TRYING

TRYING: LOVE, LOOSE PANTS AND THE QUEST FOR A BABY

Summersdale Publishers Ltd
46 West Street
Chichester
West Sussex
PO19 1RP
UK

www.summersdale.com

Printed and bound by CPI Group (UK) Ltd, Croydon, CR0 4YY

ISBN: 978-1-84953-398-0

TRYING

LOVE, LOOSE PANTS & THE QUEST FOR A BABY

MARK COSSEY

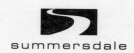

summersdale

Contents

Part 3: Try Hard with a Vengeance

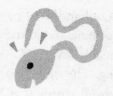

Prologue

Masturbatum Contra Mundum

'Here again, Mr Cossey?' asked the young Spanish embryologist, shooting me a welcoming smile as I followed him down the corridor. He had recognised me by sight and that wasn't good. I was now the one thing you don't want to be in a fertility clinic.

A regular.

'Here again,' I agreed, enthusiasm stapled across my face as we shuffled past various women going through various stages of not getting pregnant. I was desperately trying to maintain an air of virile, energetic masculinity, but the truth was I was knackered: partly because of encroaching middle age, partly because I had spent the previous night in the bath getting divorced.

The whole thing had been, at least partially, Martha's fault; she was the one who first brought up the subject. She was the one who sat on the cold tiles of our bathroom floor, fiddling with her wedding ring, a handful of pasta pesto I had thrown at her congealing in her hair, and asked:

'What about an amicable divorce?'

We had been fighting. The fight had been triggered by the worst words in the world; words that had dogged us for the last few years, words that Martha had uttered an hour before, in tears, during the ad break of *Location, Location, Location.*

'I just want,' she had said, 'a baby.'

These were the words tearing us apart.

Of course the whole idea of a polite break-up was ridiculous. For starters, Martha and I couldn't argue amicably about anything. We were the most incompetent arguers ever. We couldn't even fight about normal couply things: our biggest disagreement up to this point had been about the number of dimensions a cloud has. Three, by the way. Clouds, like every other object in the universe, have three dimensions. Not two. Nothing with mass has only two dimensions. It's infuriating.

But that night even the cloud argument seemed like a fond memory. This fight was different. This was about us being an infertile couple and whether or not we could survive that fact. This was bigger than the clouds.

I lay in the bath, lit a Marlboro Red and drew deeply. It seemed as good a time as any to take up smoking again. Then I tried to think of an answer to Martha's question...

Then I was back at the clinic.

'This time we have better luck, no?' The Spaniard patted my shoulder manfully, guiding me closer to my fate.

Luck. I wondered if my reproductive organs could, for once, find some. My brain and penis were already united in their opposition to producing anything that day. In fact, they had made it clear that if I wanted to see any action in the sperm-producing department, I'd better find them better working conditions.

'We're not fourteen,' they chorused. 'We're forty. We need comfort, privacy, access to your wife and/or the Internet. For pity's sake, we can't just *put out* in an NHS hospital. Gone are the glory days, the days when just being near a lingerie catalogue gave us an erection, when sitting on a bus sent us into orgasmic delight.' 'Gone', clanged the bells of my masculine doom, 'gone'.

They were right, of course, but this wasn't about me anymore. For the sum total of our married life, Martha and I had been descending into the painful, humiliating and surreal world of people who are childless but don't want to be. We had watched our friends start their families. We had been misunderstood, shouted at, pitied – and I wasn't sure which was worse. Martha had been prodded, scanned, stabbed, inseminated, overstimulated, and gone through the menopause. We had discovered the meaning of the word 'ferning'. All in our desire to have a baby.

So it didn't matter that I felt about as frisky as a eunuch who'd slept in a bath or that work kept calling me about something to do with sheep and a TV presenter, without any clarity about which sheep and what had gone wrong whilst filming them. It didn't matter that Martha had walked out earlier that morning without saying a word. Today none of that mattered. Today I just had to produce sperm – potent, healthy sperm. The future existence of my family depended on it.

We stopped outside a door. There was no sign, but I knew what lay behind that beech veneer. Every man who has ever

gone down the road of a medically assisted pregnancy knows.
It didn't need a name and anyway what would you call it?
A masturbatory? The ejaculatum? I wondered what happened
when the architects met to discuss a new clinic:

'Right, we've got the theatre, recovery, the labs, reception...
hey, what's this little room here?'
  'Where?'
  'Just next to the toilets.'
  'Oh, nothing.'
  'Nothing?'
  'Well, you know it's... for men.'
  'For men?'
  'You know, to do men's stuff.'
  'Men's stuff?'
  'Yep.'
  'And we don't have a name for that?'
  'It's just men's stuff.'
  'We could call it the phall...'
  'Look, no one really wants to talk about it, OK?'

The room's furnishings followed the same, don't-mention-the-
W-word philosophy. The spartan table and chair assumed that
any man can and will achieve orgasm under any conditions
short of a sustained artillery assault. That every man has the
power to conjure up an erection purely from the memory of
Samantha Thomson's breasts in the sixth form.

On one side was an en suite bathroom to 'clean yourself
up afterwards' as one of the female embryologists had put
it. What did she think happened? Some kind of uncontrolled

explosion? Did other men create a post-ejaculatory mess of such biblical proportions that they needed a wash?

I must have been a disappointment. Indeed, I'm positive she sighed each time she was faced with my modest efforts, holding up my samples as if to say: 'Come on, Mr Cossey, is that it?' To which the answer should have been 'Yes, it fucking is', but then you can't piss off the embryologists. Who knows what revenge they might wreak?

No, when a young, blonde, female sperm-expert examines your finest efforts with a disparaging frown, it's best to walk away with what's left of your tail between your legs.

Mercifully, this time I had the Spaniard who surely had a clearer grasp of the process involved. He motioned me into the purgatorial chamber.

'Don't forget to lock,' he said.

They said that every time. Maybe it was part of their training, maybe they were tested on it. 'Should the door to the wankatorium be locked or unlocked? Discuss in 500 words or less.'

Maybe they said it because it is the kind of thing you're likely to forget when attempting to self-stimulate in a public place. Who wouldn't leave the door slightly ajar whilst coaxing their uncooperative member into life? They've seen it all before, right? Well, except that blonde one. I'm not sure what she'd seen before; had she been conducting fertility experiments on her boyfriend? Turning him into some kind of terrifying penile fire hose?

I assured the Spaniard that the door would be sealed before my phallus greeted the fluorescent lights of the clinic. He nodded, then he paused a minute. Then he gave a small tut. He stroked his goatee beard. Finally he pointed at a black folder resting on the side table.

'The magazines,' he announced, as if heralding the arrival of Hannibal Lecter for dinner. His tanned, chiselled face seemed to blush. Once again I mused: why mention this? It was not beyond me to work out what was inside the sole unmarked folder in a room where men came to 'do their business'.

Maybe they didn't have pornography in Spain? Or was English porn, like its cuisine, too stodgy and tasteless for his Latin blood? His expression gave away nothing.

'I know,' I mumbled, attempting to share his shame about the folder.

'Of course,' he shrugged. 'You are, how do we say it, a regular.'

Then he left me to it. Embryologists, I've noticed, never shake hands.

I stood still for a moment. He was right. I did know all about it. I knew about 'Club Hardcore' and 'Big Ones' and 'Amateur Housewives'. I'd spent too long in that room; long enough to see the NHS refresh and replace their selection of Britain's worst dirty magazines many times. Long enough to know exactly which material the St William's Trust were inclined towards and what tastes were catered for. Long enough to wonder why 'Swedish Schoolgirls' had been removed from the list.

Two years, I thought, picking up the black folder. Two long years I had known this room. I locked the door and then I was alone.

My back ached. I wished I hadn't actually slept in the bath. I wished I had slept on the sofa like any other normal idiot. Most of all, I wished I had slept in the bed with Martha, but that would have been impossible. The argument had gone too far. Back in the bathroom she'd sat up and was attempting to remove the remaining pasta from her scalp with a hairbrush.

'You really want a divorce?' I asked, studying her face in the mirror; but she simply looked into the air intensely, her lips slightly pursed, her breathing shallow.

'I just…' But she couldn't finish the sentence. She couldn't say the words that had started the argument. She couldn't say them because they were the worst words in the world.

But I could hear them, and they cut through me.

'Fine,' I shouted. 'But it won't be amicable. It will be the worst divorce in the history of divorces ever. It will be the 9/11 of divorces. I will take divorce to a new level!'

'A new level?' she snapped. 'Will it be a Level 7 Wizard divorce? Will you slay the divorce dragons with your +5 divorcing mace?'

This was unfair. I grew up in a small town and there was nothing else to do except play Dungeons and Dragons. I kept the manuals purely for sentimental and investment purposes.

'At least I can have a child when I'm seventy!' I shouted.

It was a dirty, low blow. Martha paused a moment, then threw the brush at me and stormed out of the room. I slumped further into the bath and smoked my Marlboro and realised that, once again, it was just possible I had overreacted. We had no idea why we couldn't have a child. Like so many couples our infertility was unexplained. It could be her, it could be me, it could be the combination of both of us, but that just seemed to make the whole thing worse: theoretically a baby could turn up at any time.

It just hadn't.

And now Martha was lying in the other room sobbing over the state of our marriage. How had it come to this?

I pushed the scene out of my mind – this was not the time to think of Martha crying, or the bath, or those terrible words.

This was the time to wank.

The aim of my visit, if you haven't quite clocked on yet, was simple: to arouse myself, masturbate, and shoot/scrape/in some way deliver my sperm into a 50-ml specimen jar and then deliver this effort to the embryologist. Later my sperm would be introduced to Martha's eggs and then maybe, just maybe, the heavens would smile on us and give us what we were so desperate for: a baby. For that to happen, it was critical I got this ejaculation right.

Of course how to achieve an accurate ejaculation is never explained. No instructions are ever printed out, you are just expected to know what to do. You are asked for 'a sample' on the assumption that you know what kind of sample to produce and how to package it into a small plastic container.

It's not a big thing, this jar. You could miss. Professionals do. Male porn stars (I've heard) are always missing whatever it is they're supposed to hit, and yet I'm sure they don't have to crawl around afterwards, cleaning up their mess and hoping no one notices. And when they do miss they probably get some kind of on-the-job training, and everyone in the production says, 'Don't worry about it, Mr Guy Norm-Ass, happens to the best of us.'

In short, I imagine they get some guidance on the matter of how to aim sperm.

Not in the NHS. If I missed, I was on my own. There was no one to tell me what to do; did I clean it up off the ground and hope that no one noticed? Was that hygienic? Did I tell someone that I'd 'lost' my contribution to a £5,000 operation because at the crucial moment my mobile went off, sending my potential firstborn all over 'Lesbian Lovers' and that strangely absorbent shirt I happened to be wearing?

Did I ask for another go? Sadly I couldn't – I'd have been saving this lot up in my testicles for days to maximise the quantity and quality of my 'output'. I would have been under strict instructions to bring in a big cheery load of happy, healthy sperm, not some sloppy seconds because I found it difficult to aim.

Meanwhile, out in reception, Martha had probably arrived, still upset and angry, her ovulation pinpointed to a single hour of this specific morning by a month-long regime of drugs, scans, pokes and probes. Success rested on a few well-placed millilitres of uncooperative goo. Miss, and I would destroy months of painful and expensive work, add to the years of heartache, and put the future of my bloodline at risk. Miss, and I would let down my wife, my family, and deny my own child its very existence.

Miss? You don't miss.

I pushed these thoughts out of my mind, sat down, and tried to relax. Then it came back to me: the chair. The anti-wank chair. The armchair designed to stop you getting any kind of angle where gravity might assist you with the job in hand. The chair which ensures that your container remains upside down at all times, so even if you somehow hit the mark, your sperm will simply dribble back down the sides.

I wriggled around and tried some new positions, undiscovered in my decades-long exploration of the masturbatory arts, but the anti-wank chair had been designed by some kind of genius: a shadowy figure whose love of chairs was only matched by his desire to prevent the continuation of the human species.

Another thought crept into my mind. I wondered how many of my fellow ejaculators had sat on that very chair, and how many arses, au naturel, had touched the cheap fabric before I'd rested my sorry butt on it. My mind became full of the endless number of sweaty male posteriors that had shuffled, squirmed and squatted on this de Sade-inspired piece of furniture, desperate to find some workable position.

With a Herculean effort, I forced these thoughts from my mind. I picked up the container, grasped my shrivelled manhood and tried to open a well-thumbed magazine. Then I thought: how long do I have? All eternity seemed too short, yet I knew that back in reception there were a dozen other men waiting for their own turn in this little piece of hell. No pressure, I told myself, no pressure. And for a while there was no pressure. Anywhere.

More time passed. I began to panic; I frantically peeled back the pages of 'Teenage Teasers' in a vain attempt to entice my reproductive organ back to life. Then, in a final *coup d'état* my brain reminded me that, at this very moment, maybe fifty people knew exactly what I was doing.

They knew because this is the only time during the treatment of infertility that the man gets called up on his own. By name. Ten minutes before I had sat there, in the waiting room, with the other women and their other halves, with a few nurses, reception staff, the odd doctor and the bloke who empties the bins. I had read my paper and texted and just prayed for an Immaculate Conception, anything to get my mind off what I was about to do.

Then the Spanish embryologist had called out.

'Mr Cossey?'

I had squeezed past another couple, the woman smiling sympathetically, as if to let me know 'Look, it's none of my business, but good luck with that wank.' Her partner had raised an eyebrow, war veteran to war veteran: 'Focus on the wank, focus on the wank,' he had seemed to communicate telepathically. I had strolled past the rest of the assembled crowd, all thinking 'There goes Mr Cossey, off to have a wank. Anyone got a stopwatch?'

Then I had signed for my pygmy-sized jism jar and then I was back in the room with the magazines and the en suite bathroom. I took a deep breath and tried to ignore it all and then...my phone rang. This is the other thing you must do before a scheduled wank. Turn the phone off. Not to 'vibrate', that can cause its own problems, but 'off'. Otherwise, you'll do what I always did and pull it out to see who's calling.

It was Martha. I didn't hesitate – I was desperate to hear her voice.

'I just want a baby,' she whispered. In the background I could hear the reception filling up with other women wanting exactly the same thing.

I winced. *I just want a baby.* The worst words in the world. Of all the words ever conceived these were the most heart-wrenching, soul-destroying words in existence. They told me that the one thing Martha truly wanted I couldn't give her. If she'd wanted a Mulberry handbag or a flock of Albanian goats or democracy in North Korea, then I would have been in with a chance, but a baby?

It seemed impossible.

'I know,' I said, hearing a crack in my voice. Here was my failure laid before me. Martha was thirty-three. She still had time to find someone else, to try again. There was still time for a civilised separation. We both knew it. There was a pause, a long, long pause. I sat motionless on the anti-wank chair with my trousers around my ankles and waited for the end.

'But,' her voice trembled. 'Only with you. I don't want a baby with anyone else but you.'

The air fell out of my lungs. I bowed my head and rubbed the back of my neck. *Only with me.* The world's most incompetent domestic dispute had come to an end and the Cosseys were through it. We were back in the game, ready to face everything that was being thrown at us.

'Now,' Martha's voice was suddenly all calm and steel. 'You get going and you wank like you're wanking for England.'

I put the phone down. I stood up and punched the air and did a little victory dance. To be fair it was more of a victory shuffle due to the position of my trousers, but there was new wind in my sail now; I may have been a man with an undiagnosed fertility issue, but I had sperm, an almost perfected technique for putting it in a jar, and I wasn't getting an amicable divorce from the woman I loved. It was time to get a grip on myself. Literally. I sat down, took my penis in my hand, picked up a pornographic magazine, then put it down because the irony was I couldn't hold a magazine and a jar and self-stimulate at the same time, and then... and then I wanked.

I wanked because Martha and I desperately wanted a baby. We really did. We had been trying for forever. I felt like I'd let her down a hundred times, this woman who I'd always wanted to give everything to. I'd lived with her disappointment for months and then years. I'd seen the pain inside her eyes grow, and felt more powerless than I'd ever imagined. So, with my member finally pointing optimistically towards the ceiling, I called out to God, Fate and medical science that this time, this time we'd get lucky.

I went back to the reception and saw Martha sitting at the back, texting on her BlackBerry, biting her nails. This was our sixth round of fertility treatment, and like everyone in that waiting room, we were scared. Scared of never having a baby, scared of never being able to share the love we had with our own flesh and blood. Scared? We were terrified.

I sat down next to my wife. She took hold of my arm tightly, as if I might disappear: but I wasn't going anywhere.

'Asif Iqbal,' the Spanish embryologist called out. Mr Iqbal was sitting next to me and something about him suggested it was his first time. He got up gingerly and our eyes met. Two men, masturbating for their family's future, hoping against hope for that one simple miracle of life. We saluted each other with the wry half-smile of men going into battle for those they love.

Martha squeezed tighter on my arm. Even now she refused to bow to the fear, refused to give up, refused to let the whole thing take over her life. We were OK. We didn't know whether we would ever have a child of our own, but we knew that, whatever happened, we would get through it together. Then we settled down to do what you do most of when trying for a baby: we waited.

This is our story of infertility, how we got through it, and what it means to be a couple when one of the most fundamental things is denied to you. This is a story about despair, love and masturbation. And most of all this is the story about Jimmy, our son, who finally made it into the world thanks to Martha, medical science, and a wank in a little room out the back of St William's hospital.

PART 1

TRY HARD

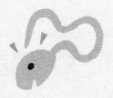

Chapter 1

Loose Pants

'It's fine,' Martha said, trying not to look me in the eye. It wasn't. I'd just carried my new wife over the threshold and already things weren't going to plan. In front of us, in the hotel's so-called honeymoon suite, were two single beds and a half-full ashtray next to the TV.

'For who?' I asked. 'Celibate smokers?'

Martha disentangled herself from my arms, sat down on one of the beds, and began to test the mattress. On the far side of the room a tropical fish tank rested precariously on a side table. Its inhabitants regarded us wearily, as though they had seen it all before.

'Come on,' she said, optimistically bouncing up and down. 'It'll be fun.'

I didn't want our wedding night to be fun. I wanted it to be perfect and this wasn't the way I imagined our nuptials being consummated. Whatever that meant. I began outlining a letter of complaint in my mind when perfection suffered another blow: something was floating at the top of the tank.

We approached the object gingerly, Martha still in her wedding dress, and studied it for a moment.

'It looks pretty dead,' Martha pronounced, sniffing the air. She was being kind; it was far beyond dead, it was decomposing. We were witnessing a dead fish rotting in its own warm bath.

'I'll sort this,' I said manfully, striding out the door, embracing with gusto the new responsibilities of a married man.

An hour later the situation remained unsorted. I had, however, managed to get caught up in the middle of a fight between the core fan base of a Scottish football team and a Korean receptionist who couldn't see what was wrong with our sleeping arrangements.

'You're lucky – you have the fish,' he assured me. 'Not everyone gets the fish.'

It was weirdly impossible to argue against this, especially with twenty middle-aged men from Aberdeen chanting something that was possibly racist. I returned shamefaced to our room, only to find my wife with another man.

'Who's he?' I asked.

'He's here about the dead thing,' Martha beamed, now dressed in jeans and a T-shirt saying 'Mrs Cossey'. 'Come on – we've got a new room.'

'Really?'

'And we've been upgraded!' she said, laughing.

And so we were. Our new room smelled clean, had a king-sized bed and, of course, an even bigger fish tank. It was also brighter than an operating theatre. What is it about lighting in hotels? You've either got the wattage of a tanning booth or a Nordic crime thriller. It's beyond me why they can't just have a single button marked, I don't know, 'lights', which allows you to either have or not have a reasonable amount of light. But no, instead you have to go on a light-switch hunt.

'You're not worrying about the lights again?' Martha asked, removing Mrs Cossey and unbuckling her belt. 'The lights are OK.'

I wasn't listening, and anyway I'd started the search now. Incentivised by the removal of clothing, I hurriedly began to dim or turn off the uplighters, table lamps, spotlights and illuminated mirrors. Even the fish tank was sent into darkness so we could have some privacy from its boggle-eyed prisoners. Eventually a faultless ambience was achieved and the rest, as they say, was history. It certainly was for the fish that had just lost power to their heated ecosystem.

'OK, Mrs Cossey?' I asked later, safe in the knowledge that we were, finally, very OK.

'Very OK, Mr Cossey,' Martha nodded. It was a perfect end to a nearish perfect day, and we had done what we'd promised ourselves: we had kicked off married life with our first attempt at trying for a baby. Already we were probably just nine months from starting our own family.

This had all been agreed three and half years before, just hours after our first kiss, on the steps of St Martin-in-the-Fields.

'We should get married,' I'd said, watching the late-night revellers milling in Trafalgar Square.

'Can we?' Martha asked, resting her head on my shoulder. 'And can we have a baby? I'd like a baby.'

'A baby,' I nodded, our lives mapped out on the London vista in front of us.

We never imagined it would require anything else to make those two things happen except us. We just assumed we would get pregnant normally. I didn't actually know what that meant, but that was all right because I was the man, and to kick off a 'normal' pregnancy I only had to get one thing right. My role could be summed up with two simple words: deliver sperm.

After that I imagined myself lying back for nine months, escaping endless birthing classes, vetoing names for my firstborn, and studying ultrasound pictures which suggested a genetic similarity to the *Moomins*. Then I would panic when the moment came, drive the wrong way to the hospital, and feign surprise when Martha didn't appear at all supportive during labour.

'Look, I thought going *up* the A25 would be quicker.'
  'I'm going to cut it off!' she would cry.
  'Then I could have moved onto the A516 and avoided the traffic. Surely you can see how that might work?'
  'I'm going to cut if off and then stick it up your...'

A few hours later I would be holding a peaceful, sleeping little baby in my arms and that would be that. Job done.

Martha's role, in contrast, was ever so slightly more involved: her body had to design and build a completely new life form from scratch, turn it into a healthy mini-human and get it to the showroom in exactly nine months – all without looking. This is why men need high-status jobs and expensive timepieces. Otherwise where would we be on a first date?

'So, what do you do?'
  'Create life.'
  'Wow. Kind of like a god.'

Long uncomfortable silence.

'And you?'

'Delivery man.'

Because of this imbalance in the distribution of labour, men and women think about fertility differently. Or rather women actually do think about it, which is what Martha was doing one sunny April afternoon, four months into married life, as we lay on our bed, happily content with yet another successful 'delivery'.

'Do you think we have a problem?' she said, staring up at the ceiling.

Contentment ran off. What problem? How could there possibly be a problem? Had I lost my job? Had Martha been faking orgasms? Cancer? Did we have collective cancer? Was it possible to have collective cancer?

'You know, a problem having a baby,' she continued, putting on her glasses to emphasise the seriousness of the question. I relaxed. Contentment returned, apologising for the sudden departure. I knew my wife was a creative sort and was prone to having a so-called 'imagination'. I also knew, as a man, that this concern was unnecessary. Infertility was something that happened to other people.

'Roo,' I said.

Yes, OK, we have pet names. Our pet names for each other are 'Roo' and 'Boo', though after ten years together it's still not clear who's Roo and who's Boo. We are working on that.

'Boo,' I said. 'We've been trying for all of four months. We just need to be patient.'

'Hmm,' she nodded, which was the international sign for Martha not being patient. Then she turned towards me and out of nowhere produced a three-pack of Marks and Spencer's finest boxer shorts. I studied this new arrival thoughtfully.

'These are too big,' I said, handing them back. I didn't have *that* much of middle-age spread.

'I know. It's to help your motility,' she replied.

'My mobility?'

'Motility – you know what motility is, don't you?'

This is the problem with women. You think you're having a conversation about, say, ill-fitting underwear, but turns out you're actually discussing testicular biology, a subject which had never come up in the four years we had shared the same bed.

Martha explained that the Internet had told her that sperm motility was the key to getting pregnant and that a more comfortable fit around the male genitalia would assist this.

'You could also consider a looser cut of trouser,' she went on.

'Like MC Hammer?'

'Worked for him.'

You couldn't argue with the evidence. MC Hammer's trousers could house a Bedouin tribe and he's had five kids – despite telling everyone they can't touch it.

I wore the pants. For the sake of my wife, some dodgy science, and the cotton industry, I spent the first part of every morning looking like Sinbad on a beach holiday, and this was our first tentative step in a long struggle to have a baby. Those pants were a symbol of a battle that starts with loose boxer shorts and ends with the illegal purchase of a child in China. Loose underwear was a Rubicon crossed: Martha and I had entered the world of assisted conception.

Sadly the pants strategy proved ineffective. Both as undergarments and as fertility enhancers, they were useless.

Two more months passed and Martha was still not pregnant. I began to notice other changes around the flat.

'Why,' I shouted one morning from the loo, 'is my 1997 copy of *Wisden* buried under a pile of pregnancy tests?'

'Got to be sure,' Martha shouted back. Sure? I wondered. Wouldn't it become obvious soon enough? Surely nature had its own ways of letting you know a baby was on its way?

'Just look at the Argos catalogue,' she chirped. That seemed to have survived the invasion, I noted. I didn't want to read the Argos catalogue. I didn't like the Argos catalogue. I calmed myself; if it helps us get a baby, I thought, then let's read the damn catalogue. I opened the bible of shopping onto garden furniture.

Around this time Martha also started coming to bed shivering with extreme cold. She would crawl under the duvet, her teeth chattering, and nuzzle up to me.

'Are you sick?' I asked.

'C-cold bath,' she shivered.

'Cold bath?'

'Just a pr-pr-precaution…'

Eventually she admitted that she had read somewhere (i.e. the Internet again) how hot baths could cause embryos to spontaneously die. Or explode or something, I can't remember the details, but the result was that for the next two weeks Martha went without hot water, all in the hope of getting pregnant.

'You don't think I'm overreacting, do you?' she asked one night, mentally preparing herself for the bath ahead.

I didn't know how to respond. To be honest, I thought she was crackers, but in a sweet, superficial and endearing way.

'Er…'

'You do think I am!' she cried, shocked. 'You think I'm overreacting.'

This happened sometimes. Martha would respond to my underreaction to her overreaction by overreacting. I called it the double overreact. There was, of course, the triple-overreact, but that's a different story. The double required a careful, diplomatic touch to stop things spiralling out of hand.

'Roo, shut up,' I said. Martha stared at me, as if about to pounce, then put her head in my lap and stared at the TV.

'I'm not overreacting,' she sniffed. 'I just want us to have a baby.'

'We will,' I said emphatically, changing the channel. An aging Captain Kirk was fighting Malcolm McDowell on some cheap film set.

'Us not having a baby,' I continued, 'would be like Captain Kirk dying and the Enterprise blowing up. We're destined for it.'

Martha was momentarily reassured by my conviction, so it was frustrating when five minutes later the Enterprise blew up and Captain Kirk died. You just can't trust anything anymore.

Despite the impeccable scientific principle behind the cold-bath theory, Martha remained without child. It didn't worry me, I was still heavily sceptical of the need for any assistance or self-help, confident that sooner or later one of my 'deliveries' would naturally find its way to one of her eggs. Then, before I knew it, I would be feeling the thrill of a correctly sized waistband once again.

This all changed at a friend's party in August. Martha and I had been married for eight months when we walked into the already humming, slightly over-lit flat and made a beeline for two old friends.

'Are you trying yet?' one asked suddenly.

The question came out of the blue. Was it obvious? Did people not using birth control have a certain look?

'Well…' Martha blushed.

'I bet you're getting it,' Friend Number Two winked at me.

'What?'

'You know – sex. I bet it's on tap in your house.'

I wondered whether other people remained chaste until deciding to have a baby. Also, wasn't it just bad manners to inquire how much sex I was or was not getting? Still, I didn't want to appear rude.

'It is flowing quite freely,' I confessed with mock pride.

'So you *are* trying,' nodded Friend Number One.

I'd always thought getting married was a mixture of tax efficiency and an overpriced romantic gesture, but no: it turns out when you sign those forms you also declare that everyone now has a stake in your sex life. Everyone: friends, strangers, their mums, your sister. Why is beyond me. Friend Number Two inched closer.

'The thing is,' he winked, 'me and Sam are thinking of having a go ourselves soon.'

There was a pause. What was I meant to say?

'So,' he continued. 'Got any advice?'

Have sexual intercourse? Don't wear a condom by accident? I didn't know how to reply – the last time I had this intimate a conversation about sex I was fourteen and playing a game that involved two oat biscuits. You don't want to know. I began to imagine an alternative universe where such conversations were commonplace.

'So are you trying?' I would ask.

'What, for a baby?' replied alternative-universe Friend Number Two.

'No, an orgasm. Are you trying for an orgasm? I've been trying for years.'

'To be honest, we've gotten a bit stuck on penetration.'

'I'm actually a virgin.'

'I'm prepubescent.'

'I've got crabs!' I retorted cleverly.

It was then that I realised that half the party were listening to me and my alternative-universe conversation where I had, for reasons unknown, given myself a sexually transmitted disease. Not for the first time, I made a mental note to keep things in my own head in future, and not to pretend I was infected in a social situation.

Martha pulled me out on to the roof terrace. The evening was quiet – just a few people smoking cigarettes, watching the sun set, listening to a distant siren. Then we noticed the Skeletors.

The Skeletors were a married couple we vaguely knew. Unfortunately for them they looked a bit like Skeletor and the kind of woman Skeletor might marry – if Skeletor was into women, which I doubt. I imagined he was probably in the closet.

'Ha ha ha. I've got you trapped, He-man. Your only escape is to wrestle me to the ground!'

'We've done that at least fifteen times, Skeletor.'

'Really?'

'Uh-huh – and can we stop with the old "sword in your pocket" routine…'

Back on the terrace Mrs Skeletor seemed to be having her own epiphany, and was arguing bitterly with her husband.

'You said you'd stop boozing this time.'

'What difference does it make?'

'Do you actually want this? Do you?'

Martha explained the Skeletors' misery later that evening, in the cab home.

'Fourth round of IVF,' she said. I'd vaguely heard of IVF, but had no idea what it entailed; only that it had something to do with helping couples have babies.

'Apparently they're not happy,' she continued, a little worried frown on her face.

Of course they weren't happy. They couldn't have a child. They looked like skeletons. Was Martha worried about looking like a skeleton? I got the cab to stop at a McDonald's and, two Big Macs later, things seemed a little cheerier. Martha sipped at her Coke and sighed.

'We're on the clock now,' she said. I understood. Now other people knew we wanted a baby. It shouldn't have made a difference, but somehow it mattered and suddenly a little bit of pressure slipped into the bedroom.

We reached eight months of 'trying' and Martha was still without child. Even I had begun to think, 'Where's this baby, then?' and wondered whether or not there might be something wrong with us. Overnight, a small gremlin installed himself in the Cossey household.

'Have you noticed we've got a gremlin?' I asked.

'He's been here for months,' shrugged Martha.

We tried to be realistic. Medical experts will tell you to wait at least a year before worrying. Even two years' delay is not unusual. Just relax and keep doing what you're doing, they will say. But how do they know what you're doing? You could be doing it wrong. You could literally be buggering the whole thing up, couldn't you?

What these experts didn't understand is that Martha and I had trouble waiting ten minutes. For anything. Waiters, check-ins, eclipses – we just didn't have it in us to be patient. Martha and I had been brought up to believe conception was easier and more likely than catching an infectious disease in a British hospital.

Martha and I also coped with frustration in different ways. My technique involved puffin-clubbing. No, this was not me letting my hair down in some Ibizan discotheque. This was me shouting threats to club puffins. This was because I assumed God wouldn't allow such a thing and therefore would give me what I wanted. God doesn't like anyone going after puffins, that's why he made them so cute. Martha, on the other hand, had a different strategy: in the face of adversity she took action. I knew something was coming, mainly because the house gremlin had been in a panic for days, furiously gesticulating at my watch and sending me meeting requests on my phone. Nonetheless, it was still a surprise when Martha came home one night and announced solemnly:

'We're getting a calendar.'

Before 'The Calendar' arrived, the Julian system held no menace for me. It was all good stuff – how many days to

Christmas? When's my birthday? What holidays are coming up next? A calendar was a friend, a keeper of time, guardian of the weekend.

Then The Calendar turned up. It appeared on the fridge door, with a little cross marked against the seventeenth. That cross changed things forever.

This was Calendargate.

At first the date meant nothing to me. The next morning I considered The Calendar over a cup of tea. What trouble could a few pieces of numbered card cause? Surely this was no more than loose pants in laminate form, and yet there was something faintly sinister about it all, something I couldn't quite put my finger on.

My musings were interrupted by a rumbling below and I shuffled off to the toilet. I picked up the Argos catalogue and opened it to page thirty-seven. While it was no replacement for my buried *Cricketers' Almanack*, I was now finding the book curiously addictive. I already had my eye on a See-saw Meerkat Garden Ornament for the window box.

Then I noticed something else. The pregnancy tests had been pushed slightly to one side to make way for a new tower of boxes. I picked one of them up and studied the packaging.

It read: *Ovulation testing kit – 95% accurate.*

Back then I was ignorant about the reproductive innards of my wife, so when Martha got home that evening my principle concern was that the toilet's original function – i.e. as a sacred place of male meditation – was now in jeopardy due to its new role as a storage depot for Boots. What man could relax on his own bog with this sinister array of fertility pharmaceuticals next to him?

And what was an ovulation testing kit anyway?

'It tests for when you ovulate,' Martha said.

Silence. Martha puffed her cheeks and blew air.

'You do know what ovulation is, don't you?'

I did recall something from school about an over rate of a follicle in hyperspace, but it seemed the wrong moment to bring this up. Martha sat me down. Using small words, she explained that she was only fertile a few days during each month and it was only during this small window that my sperm had any chance of finding her egg and making us a baby. She then went on to explain that my sperm could only survive in her for about a day, what with the antibodies in her vagina wanting to kill them and the exhausting, Byzantine path they needed to follow to reach her egg.

'And then my egg might just reject you,' she continued, hammering yet another nail into the Darwinian theory of evolution. What was this, I thought. Survival of the most complicated reproductive system? A Japanese game show? It's like you go all the way across town with a nice bottle of Jacob's Creek and then Miss Egg just wants to watch *An Affair to Remember* and tell you what a good friend you are.

'... and even if your sperm does manage to fertilise the egg, often the embryo just self-aborts naturally.'

Suicidal embryos. We were up against suicidal embryos.

'So,' she finished, 'can you see why I'm worried?'

I nodded and slumped deeper into our sofa. How in the hell did anyone ever get pregnant?

Martha dragged me to the fridge door where The Calendar hung, waiting. She pointed at the date marked in red.

'That is when I'm likely to be most fertile. That is our best chance to get pregnant.'

I now realised the significance of The Calendar. I considered the date earnestly. Something – there was something about the seventeenth. It was on the tip of my tongue, but what was it...?

'That,' I said, 'is Richard's stag do.'

And that was when our first fertility fight started.

In retrospect I accept that my firstborn, conceived or not, should have taken priority over Richard's stag. I accept it was unreasonable to refuse a compromise involving a fleeting appearance by Martha during the festivities, and how frustrating it must have been to find her husband prioritising a piss-up on the Welsh borders over trying to start a family.

'But we're sharing a room at the Ibis,' I cried.

Martha suggested that Richard and I might want to make this arrangement permanent. That I could consider an immediate move to the hotel, and not bother waiting for the seventeenth. I replied by agreeing that living with Richard might be for the best, that at least he accepted me for me and didn't go on about some cereal bowl which I occasionally failed to put *in* the dishwasher.

'I leave it nearby,' I protested.

'It doesn't wash things *near* it.' Martha threw up her arms.

To be honest, I wasn't convinced Richard and I would have a happy life together, but Martha didn't understand: while men only have a single function in the whole reproductive business, they are also completely rubbish at it. For example, men can't schedule. They will deliver, but not to a schedule.

That night, having forestalled my emigration to the Ibis, I went onto the Internet to see what all this infertility fuss was about. I still didn't take the whole thing too seriously, and I still thought it was all a bit hysterical getting so worried about having a baby. Conception, I reasoned, would happen in its own good time.

Not on the World Wide Web it doesn't. On forum after forum, I discovered all the heart-wrenching, gut-turning stories of couples who had been trying for years to have children to no avail. Couples who had lost whole decades of their lives, and would spend decades more coming to terms with this cruel denial of their desire to reproduce.

I didn't bother with the fact that, despite all these stories, most women do get pregnant. Oh no. Eight months in and I went straight for the jugular. Reading about Haley from Texas, whose husband left her after six years of infertility treatment and now won't let her touch the remaining embryos, even though he'd now managed a family of four with a pole dancer from Austin.

I realised this was the world Martha had been living in. I had always assumed her time online had been full of emails, shopping, and waiting for Friends Reunited to be replaced with something good. Now, examining our Internet history, I found a world of fear, full of horrible stories of women's broken dreams.

I had no choice: I either had to become a slightly better husband or destroy the Internet.

I went back into our bedroom and lay down next to my wife, who was reading quietly.

'What's that?' I asked.

She lifted the book so I could see the cover. It read *The Fastest Way to Get Pregnant Naturally*.

'Any help?'

Martha raised an eyebrow sceptically. Then I noticed one of the doors to our wardrobe had been opened. Inside was the stuffed toy seal we had bought optimistically on our honeymoon. A sheet had been neatly placed over it, hiding it from view.

'Sorry,' I said.

Martha put down her book on her lap. I sat next to her on the bed.

'It's all right, I shouldn't be so paranoid. You go.'

'To the Ibis? I said I was sorry.'

'To the stag do!'

She snuggled in under my shoulder. For a while we just looked out the window of our flat, watching the last remains of sunlight fade.

'I'm thirty in a couple of weeks,' Martha said finally. 'I always thought I'd be pregnant before thirty.'

I began to stroke her hair until eventually her breathing told me she had fallen asleep. Then I looked down at my manhood, also snoozing comfortably beneath its gigantic pants, and sighed. The Internet was too big to be deleted.

'Well fella,' I whispered, 'looks like we're going to have to schedule.'

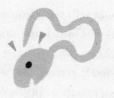

Chapter 2

The Schedule

Martha's birthday passed with much pomp and celebration, and now the stage was set for the seventeenth. For the first time ever we were planning our sex life to coincide with her ovulation. We were nervous and impatient and the tension was heightened by the introduction of a sex curfew three days before the big night.

'A sex what?' I asked, staring at my wife.

'We need to optimise your sperm count,' Martha smiled, patting me on the knee. 'So no masturbation either.'

I looked over towards The Calendar. Once she's pregnant, I thought, that calendar is going to die. I made a mental note to buy matches.

The evening before, our lives moved at their usual frantic pace. Martha, like me, was a TV producer, and she was currently working with *EastEnders* on a night shoot somewhere in north London. I was trapped in a Cardiff club with hundreds of crazed *Doctor Who* fans.

'It's for your own safety,' shouted the bouncer, blocking the exit. Outside, the sound of approaching sirens began to overwhelm the eighties pop mix.

'We're with the Doctor!' we shouted back. The bouncer shook his head. Even a Time Lord couldn't survive Church Street on a Friday night.

By the time the day itself arrived we were exhausted. Neither of us had managed more than a couple of hours' sleep and this, along with the enforced celibacy, had left us more than a little sensitive. In retrospect, it was therefore a bad idea to spend the afternoon in IKEA.

Perhaps we were hoping that a discussion about the dimensions of a Kumbfort sofa would distract us from the crucial evening ahead. It did not. We disagreed strongly about the Kumbfort. When I say 'disagreed', I mean we fought. About what, only the gods of self-assembly remember, but we left the store with a lot of bad karma, a ladle and some tea lights bouncing around in the back of our hired minivan.

Why do couples go to IKEA? No love, not Romeo and Juliet, not Abelard and Héloïse, not Posh and Becks, could survive the IKEA experience. Orwell didn't imagine a boot stamping on a human face forever – he just went to IKEA for some kitchen utensils and saw it for real.

The combination of shopping, Cardiff and *EastEnders* hadn't left us in the most amorous mood, but we were good fertility soldiers. Agreeing never to enter a Swedish home-furnishing store together again, we kicked off our journey into planned sex as ordained by the ovulation test and The Calendar.

To help us, Martha had read some fertility books. In each one there was always a chapter on 'romance', full of useful hints on how to get your partner relaxed and in the mood for sex. I'm not sure who writes these books, but their idea of a romantic evening was not mine. One suggested that 'dinner and a show' was the perfect way to get ready for procreational activity, as though all couples lived within commuting distance of Broadway or the West End.

And had this expert ever tried doing it after a dodgy pre-theatre meal followed by two and a half hours of *Les Misérables*?

'Shall we, you know, hop in the sack?'

'I'd love to, but I can't get that boy being shot dead out of my head.'

'I keep hearing Susan Boyle.'

'OK, just let me go to the toilet. I shouldn't have had the lamb rogan josh...'

Another book recommended jigsaws. Yes, jigsaws as a way to prepare for sex. But how can you relax doing a jigsaw? For those that do, I can only ask: why? You know how it's going to turn out. It's printed on the front of the box. You could just put the box on your table and look at that.

Was it even a good thing to be relaxed when attempting conception? Niger has one of the highest birth rates in the world and it isn't the kind of place you'd go to for a romantic mini-break. I can't imagine musicals feature strongly in their lovemaking rituals:

'We're trying for a baby.'

'You relaxing? You need to relax.'

'Yeah, after I've finished the civil war, we're going to take in the locust plague and watch any surviving crops wilt in the horrendous heat.'

'Not trying a jigsaw then?'

Thankfully, romance was a different beast in the Cossey household. There were to be no cardboard-based puzzles or trips to *Starlight Express* for us. I had already planned the ultimate romantic schedule: Thai takeaway and a bottle of wine, followed by a pre-recorded quarter-final match of *University Challenge*. The full seductive malarkey was laid on to get us into the frisky spirit of things.

After Martha had beaten me, answering seven questions to my three, and Paxman had bid us goodnight, we sat silently on our sofa. I waited for Martha to move. Martha waited for me to move.

'You ready?' I asked.

'Yep,' Martha's voice was a pitch higher than normal. 'You?'

'Sure,' I said looking ahead into space. 'Couldn't be readier.'

I didn't feel ready. Something felt different. Like things were going to be different. Like sex was going to be different. And by different, I mean worse.

We shuffled off to the bedroom with a slight air of embarrassment. We undressed, lay on the bed with an awkwardness new to both of us and began our attempt to 'make love'. At first we both tried to make a good fist of it. Well, not literally of course. I mean, that wouldn't help at all, would it? Or would it?

We continued at what I can only describe as fumbling foreplay underneath the best glow two Exthorp lamps could provide. We groped like two drunken teenagers on a park bench, and all the time, going around in my head was a voice complaining: '... must we do it now? Well, we could do it tomorrow morning, God, no, got to go filming at six and I haven't even ironed a shirt, in fact what shirt should I wear? AM I FIRING BLANKS? No, no, no, I'm sure it's fine, now come on, let's get down to business. Business? Like a male prostitute? If so, I need to learn how to get an erection on demand. Blanks, blankety, blankety blank... hang on, is that a baby crying somewhere?'

Suddenly a barbershop quartet – consisting of Paxman, The Gremlin, that dead kid from *Les Mis* and Skeletor – appeared at the end of the bed. They began to sing (to the tune of the classic Louis Prima version of 'Just a Gigolo'):

> *It's just a piccolo*
> *And everywhere it goes*
> *People ask the part it's playing*
> *Stick it in loose pants*
> *It's still shooting blanks*
> *Oooh, what they saying?*
> *Now there's come a night*
> *When it won't stand upright*
> *What'll they say about it?*
> *When the end comes, you know*
> *You've got just a piccolo*
> *And you can't ejaculate without it*
> *Cause yoooooooooouuuu ain't got a baby...*

I sat up, swung my legs onto the edge of the bed, and put on my boxer shorts. I stood up. The shorts fell to the floor. This was not how I had expected the evening to go – it was as though my own mind, plus gravity, were working against me.

My imagination wasn't the only enemy. Intercourse was also being hampered by that other useless part of male psyche: the ego. I've said that men don't like being told when to have sex, but the truth is we hate it. We don't mind it being offered to us, we don't mind asking for it; some men will even try to demand it. But we will not be told.

Men like to imagine themselves so fantastic – so covered in musky sexual prowess – that at any particular moment they might choose to have sex with any number of willing nubile wenches, or they might just choose to watch highlights of the world darts championship with a can of beer resting on their belly. Evidence may suggest the time is right to try for that baby. Common sense may dictate that you should make hay while she's ovulating; but if it dents that male sense of self-importance, forget about it.

Eventually, I managed to convince my own ego that we needed to get back on the horse. OK, that's a terrible metaphor but imagine it's a very attractive horse and I'm a stallion and the whole thing is taking place in some very upmarket stables. Anyway, I stepped out of my loose pants and hopped back into the marital bed. This wasn't about fun. Or horses. This was about making a baby.

Martha was staring at me. She had been staring for some time.

'Were you just comparing me to a horse?' she said.

I really, really needed to stop thinking aloud.

'You're not…' A little doubt crawled into her voice. 'You're not going off me?'

'What?'

'You know, because I'm not pregnant. Some men go off their wives if they're having problems.'

'I'll show you how off I've gone,' I said, taking Martha into my arms and locking her in a carnal embrace. Sadly, though, while I had now become a reconstructed, civilised, loving machine, my penis had not. It was the same self-serving bastard it had always been, and it was not cooperating.

Women don't understand what it's like, having a penis. They assume it's just like any other limb. Like a hand. When you want to pick up a mug of tea with your hand, you don't even have to think about it; the hand negotiates with the arm, the fingers, et cetera, and gets that nice hot drink to your mouth without needing so much as a 'thank you'.

Penises aren't like that. For example, sometimes my penis is like having the cast of *Family Guy* strapped around my crotch. Some mornings, as I stumble off to the bathroom with a full bladder, my penis suddenly decides that now is the time to produce a rock-hard erection that could fell a Californian redwood. Why? What are the chances of having sex at 6.15 a.m., on my own, in a toilet, with a full bladder? Are those odds worth the serious discomfort caused by not being able to urinate?

'Why would your penis do that?' you ask. I don't know – I'm not my penis.

That night, however, having an erection was the last thing on its mind. Instead, it appeared to be in the penile equivalent of a vegetative coma. We tried many strange and unusual techniques to resuscitate it, but by ten to eleven the state of my manhood remained unchanged, and Martha and I were now just staring at the unhelpful fellow resting between my legs.

'This is new,' she said. It certainly was. 'Are you absolutely positive you're not going off me?'

'What should I do?' I whispered, panicking. A fear ran through me: what if this was it? What if I never had an erection again? Erectile dysfunction they called it. I had permanent erectile dysfunction. My penis seemed to shrink even more as if to confirm the prognosis.

'Can't you talk it up or something?' Martha suggested. 'It is your penis.'

Conversations with my penis rarely went well. Take the school bus in the eighth grade. Every day, without fail, an erection would occur. It was not a good place for an erection; it was, to be honest, an embarrassment. I explained this to my penis; I told it enthusiasm was, in principle, a fine thing but there was a time and a place and the bus was not it. Then, the next morning, the moment I sat down, off it went...

'Maybe,' Martha interrupted, sensing further delay. 'We could pretend we're on a bus? Would that work?'

Finally, just before the clock struck midnight, the barbershop quartet disappeared, next door's baby went to sleep and my unhelpful sexual organ finally began to stir. Then, after what was the sexual equivalent of *Star Wars: Episode 1* (highly anticipated but in the end fairly dull with a fair to middling climax), Martha and I completed our duty to continue the human race.

Then we pulled up the duvet, turned off the lights, and stared up at the ceiling. Suddenly sex had become a responsibility. Hopping into bed for a quickie had become like applying for a job, getting a mortgage, or sitting your A-levels. Except you had to do it naked. With an erection.

For the next ten days we waited anxiously to find out the outcome of our scheduled sex experiment. I was now convinced that timing was the key, and what with the ovulation test, the power of The Calendar, and the near-enough clinical insertion of my sperm, we were a shoo-in for Martha being pregnant. Finally, I thought, after seven long months we were going to begin our journey as a family.

It was a Tuesday when Martha rang me:

'It's negative,' she said.

This was a blow. We really had been 'trying' this time and it seemed unfair that all our efforts had come to nothing. I could hear the upset in Martha's voice and I wondered whether we shouldn't have been together when she did the test. I imagined my nervous wife in my arms, me like an emotional rock, telling her it would be OK, willing her to have the strength to carry on…

'What, in the toilet?' she asked. 'You want to be an emotional rock in the toilet while I piss on a stick.'

'I could stand outside,' I replied. 'And then when it's positive we could celebrate together.'

'I can't wee when someone's listening.'

Martha was slightly missing the point, I thought, though it was true that, thanks to the mountain of tests, there was no longer enough room in our loo for two people. However, having scorned them, I now understood the value of the stick. It had nothing to do with diagnostics – the most any test could do was beat nature by a few days. But it did one thing – it gave Martha control. It was the one piece of self-determination she had; choosing the moment of disappointment.

That night, when I got home, I noticed another date already marked in red pen on The Calendar. We were clearly not giving up. Sighing, I opened a bottle of wine, poured us both a glass, and raised the rim to my lips. Good old alcohol, I thought, taking a sip – there was one thing you could rely on. I looked down at my crotch indicating that it, on the other hand, had a performance issue. My crotch looked back at me and my glass of rioja and questioned whether the two might be related. I began to regret the fact that not only was I now having an argument with my own sexual organs; I also appeared to be losing it.

I turned to my wife for support, but Martha had pushed her glass to one side.

'We should cut down,' she said.

What?

'Less booze. More baby.'

What?

Martha handed me a printed-out academic paper explaining that drinking could reduce the chances of her conceiving by up to a fifth and that alcohol can affect a man's fertility as well. I began to regret the introduction of broadband to our household and the sudden influx of additional information it had brought with it. I also explained to her that if Ernest Hemingway was able to reproduce on twenty mojitos a day we should be able to manage it on half a bottle of Tesco's finest.

But Martha wasn't giving up.

'What would you rather have – wine or a baby?'

I paused to think. The thing is I love alcohol. I'm actually in love with alcohol. I began to recall all the wonderful times alcohol and I had spent together: the pubs, the beaches, the restaurants…

'Mark!' Martha pleaded.

This is how they get you. I didn't believe a word of the whole alcohol causes infertility nonsense. How many people have conceived after a drunken night on the tiles? In fact, how many people do you know who didn't have a little bit of booze swimming around their bloodstream when Mr Sperm popped off to find Ms Egg? All the evidence I had accumulated on the subject clearly proved that drinking was a crucial ingredient in the whole pregnancy thing.

Yet, thanks to some tweedy academic at Harvard, a glass of beer was now right up there in the reproductive no-go list alongside class A drug addiction and bungee jumping. I looked at the almost full bottle and then at my wife. Finally, I picked it up and unscrewed the cap.

Then I poured it down the sink.

'OK, no booze,' I agreed. Martha's shoulders relaxed and she turned back to the dinner. I stared at the empty bottle – how bad could it be, I wondered. A couple of weeks of abstinence, get the wife pregnant, then get back on the sauce. Tough, but doable.

'And we need to eat less junk,' Martha added, unhelpfully.

The only challenge was work. The thing about my job is that alcohol, like irony, is omnipresent. A week after my commitment to sobriety, I was invited to a dinner by a company who were thinking of offering me a job. It was a lavish do at a private club in west London and I had only a brief moment to take in the opulent luxury of the Georgian house before an immaculately dressed waiter offered me a cold flute of champagne.

'Water?' I asked, nervously. The waiter was visibly shocked by the request, but returned after a moment with a glass of the stuff. We both regarded it sadly, as if I was about to drink poison. I looked around; no one else was consuming anything without bubbles in it.

As we sat down to eat, I began to realise I was at a dinner the likes of which I had never known. The food was incredible; the room was held together by a giant glitter ball hanging from a curved, coloured glass dome – it was like *Brideshead* on Ecstasy. Waiters kept sliding up to me:

'Montrachet?' they would say, proffering a bottle of crisp, white wine with a golden hue.

'Water,' I croaked.

People, sensing that I was not drinking and ergo not fun, began to edge away from me.

'Mouton?' A bottle of deep, ruby-coloured red was dangled under my nose.

'Water.' Tears filled my eyes.

On it went. The dessert wine. The port. The cocktails. Everyone was having a wonderful time, everyone was completely hammered. Everyone except me. I sat there, my tenth glass of H_2O gripped manically in my hand. Then, the woman who could have been my new boss placed a hand on my shoulder.

'Not drinking?' she asked, dubiously.

I know a sober, tearful man isn't a good look but what was I to do? I had been there for four hours. Alongside the foie gras, gold-dusted turkey breast, and a dolphin-shaped pudding, I had somehow managed to eat twenty-two individual pieces of bread. My stomach and bladder were having a bloating competition inside me. I looked up at her with my moistened eyes: she was staring drunkenly down at me, Martini in hand, cigarette in the other. I had to say something.

'Water?' A waiter came in between us, holding a jug.

I was the two things you could never be in TV: sober and sober. My never-to-be boss turned away from me forever.

I slumped into my chair for a further eternity; I was an island of misery in what appeared to be the greatest sea of bacchanalian fun ever had by mankind.

Two further hours passed until, when everyone else descended on the bar, I felt I could finally make a break for the exit. Just as it came into view, an arm reached out and pulled me into a drunken embrace.

'I love you,' the complete stranger said. 'I love you and I love your work and I just love you.'

I didn't love him. I just loved alcohol and missed it. I wished I could drown the greasy-haired geek who was drooling on my shirt in a pool of ethanol and then drink it. But I couldn't. We were trying to have a baby.

This new world was further tested when the evening of our next scheduled lovemaking session arrived. Now, not only did we have to have sex-upon-which-our-future-child-depended-on, but we also had to do it sober. There was not much relaxing that night as we sat in front of our vegetarian pasta bake with purified water, listening to the sound of our tap dripping.

'We need to fix that,' Martha said eventually.

'Are you sure this is going to work?' I asked.

Martha didn't answer. She picked unhappily at a limp aubergine and we continued to sit, silently, until it became clear that neither of us were going to finish our dinner. Then we dragged ourselves off to the bedroom, and there we discovered that scheduled sex was actually qualitatively worse without the benefit of any mood-altering drugs.

Two weeks later, I paced nervously outside the toilet for the result of our hard toil and deprivation. Could we, I thought, finally be pregnant? Martha had been grumpy all week and surely that was a good sign?

The answer lay with her urine.

'How's it going,' I asked, tapping gently on the door. How long did it take to piss on a stick?

'Go away,' Martha said unhelpfully. 'I can't wee with you hanging around.'

I went and paced up and down the living room instead. Several minutes later there was the sound of the toilet flushing and Martha appeared in the doorway.

'Well?'

Martha sat down on our sofa. I sat down next to her. After a moment she shook her head. That was all she did, shake her head once and we both looked down. Then she patted my leg as if England had lost the football.

'Oh well,' she said and then she went into the kitchen.

Once again the test was negative. Once again we were not pregnant. All those wasted evenings, I thought, when I could have been, well, wasted.

Dispirited, I did what I always do in a difficult and upsetting situation: I rang our local pizza delivery service and ordered an Extra-Extra-Large Mexican Hot with extra chilli beef to be delivered ASAP.

I was anticipating a fight, expecting the no-booze, healthy eating regime to be reinforced. But there was a reason why I'd married Martha. Thirty minutes later, when I arrived home from the local minimart with the most alcoholic bottle of wine I could find, the pizza, far from being in the bin, was on a little table in front of the sofa, piping hot. Next to it sat the remote control. And next to that were two wine glasses and my wife.

I sat down. We weren't pregnant, but we did have pizza and a drink and television, and later that night we had unscheduled sex, which is always the best kind you can have.

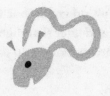

Chapter 3

Everybody's Pregnant But We Just Feel the Same

'We're having a baby!'

We sat at the dining table of Steve and Sarah Morgan, eating what appeared to be a cremated lamb. I had been concentrating on chewing the vulcanised meat, so for a moment I was unsure where the words had come from. I glanced quickly at Martha but she was silent. We weren't having a baby – the only thing we'd had was three rounds of scheduled sex and a menstrual cycle that ended two hours late. It had been a wonderful one hundred and twenty minutes but it was over now.

No, the announcement had come from our hosts.

'You're having a what?' I cried; then cried again as Martha pre-emptively kicked me in the shin. As I went down I noticed The Gremlin hiding under the table. For some reason, he had turned bright green.

'Wonderful news!' Martha cheered, raising her glass. 'We're so happy for you both.' We were? I didn't feel happy. Surprised, yes. Envious, possibly. But not happy. I stared at Steve as he manfully offered my wife another hacked-off slice of animal. What was wrong with the cooking? And what did Steve have that I didn't?

Whatever it was, it came as a shock. I had never considered the idea that other people might be trying for a baby – and worse, be better at it – but it turned out Steve and Sarah weren't alone. Within a month of the Morgans coming out three more couples announced their successful conception to us with unrestrained glee.

It was an epidemic: all around us people had caught the breeding bug. Even celebrities were at it and they're incapable of taking care of themselves. How could they possibly hope to raise a child? What were they thinking, trying to reproduce?

'I want to have a baby!'

'God, Bono, no. Remember what happened when you made poverty history.'

'I succeeded?'

'No, you triggered the biggest global recession in living memory. Please don't have a baby.'

But they all did, because a baby had become the ultimate accessory. Babies were cool. You couldn't open a copy of *Heat* magazine without some model, actress or *Big Brother* runner-up proudly displaying their bump in a bikini to the world. And if it was in *Heat* then you knew a baby boom was on its way.

Back at the Morgans I struggled with their unsettling news. My exhausted jaw continued to masticate without hope. I listened to lurid details about the risks of pregnancy; how unpasteurised cheese could kill; the chances of their offspring having Down's syndrome or Crohn's disease; or just being quite ugly to look at.

'Top up?' Steve smiled, the dimpled, handsome grin of a father-to-be. They had clearly stopped drinking, and yet hadn't hesitated to open something expensive for their guests.

Generous fertile bastards!

'We hear you two are trying,' Sarah said, thrilled by the idea. 'You'll make wonderful parents. Won't it be nice when we've all got children!'

Did everyone know? I wondered, suddenly feeling the pressure of the Morgans' verdant sexual organs nudging against mine.

Then my bladder carried me away from the table and up the stairs to the bathroom. As I stood there, relieving my physical and emotional self, I sensed something missing. An absence of certain objects. Where, I wondered, were the ovulation kits? The pregnancy tests?

Curious, I snuck into the kitchen and flipped through the past months of their calendar, but there were no marks, no dates set. Did they not have a timetable? Did they know something we didn't?

'They don't have any of the stuff we do,' I said to Martha as we walked down to the station.

'No,' she frowned.

'And yet they're pregnant.'

It began to rain.

'While you were spying on them, Sarah told me it happened first time.' Martha's frown continued as drops of water began to frizz her hair. Then The Gremlin tugged at my coat. His greenness was now luminescent.

Stupid virile Morgans, I thought. Later that evening Martha sat in front of a *Grazia* magazine sighing.

'Come on,' I said, glancing over at our bookcase. 'Why don't you read something cheery like *Tintin* or *The Bell Jar*?'

'You don't understand,' she replied, but I did. Pregnancy had become both common and fashionable. Like Zara. Ergo we had become endangered and unfashionable. Like the economic theories of North Korea. Or the kakapo, an overweight flightless bird that had been named after faeces – twice.

We were the bumbag of fecundity.

I began to grow suspicious of the loose underpants and The Calendar and the ovulation sticks. I began to wonder whether Martha had been duped by the pregnancy industry and whether I should seek understanding elsewhere. It was time to consult my fellow thirty-something males. For the truth. Surely someone would know something about it?

The following Sunday we arrived at an autumnal barbecue. A heavy shower reinforced my belief that October was a poor month for an outdoor cooking event, but, as usual, everyone invoked the Dunkirk spirit. Because that helps. The veterans of Dunkirk must get royally pissed off, their spirit being summoned each time a cloud passes over the Home Counties.

'Have you lot actually been on a beach? In northern France? Under heavy attack from the Nazis?'

'No, but feel that rain. That is wet rain. We need your spirit to carry on.'

'Have you ever heard of loose pants?' I asked my old friend Stuart, as we stood under an umbrella, burning some unhappy-looking sausages. Everyone knew he and his partner were trying for a baby.

'Moose ants? Where?' he said, lifting his barbecue implement, as if fully aware of what moose ants were, what kind of threat they possessed, and what response was required.

'No, loose pants. For the ovulating thing.'

A sausage spat at me. Stuart's expression became blank, hoping the conversation would return to the safer ground of moose ants.

'You know what ovulation is, don't you?' I pressed harder.

Stuart's face went blanker.

'No, but tell you what – did you know my ex is up the duff?'

Giving up on Stuart, I called Marv. Marv was a legend. Before he had settled down he had not only played the field, he had played all fields known to man. He had based his life philosophy on what an old Buddhist monk in Thailand had told him:

'A young bull and an old bull sit on a hill,' began the alleged monk. 'They look down at a herd of young cows. The young bull says, "Let us run down to that herd and have ourselves a cow." The old bull looks at the young bull sagely, smiles, and shakes his head. "No, let us walk down and have all of them."'

Marv had stared at me, challenging me to appreciate the depth of this ancient east-Asian wisdom.

'You see what I'm saying?' he had winked.

He wanted to have sex with a farm animal? Too much cardiovascular exercise restricts your sexual prowess? It wasn't clear.

Still, Marv was a man of the world – he was bound to know about ovulation.

'It's tricky,' I said, speaking softly into my mobile. 'I don't know who else to talk to.'

'Go to a clinic,' he shouted. He seemed to be on a train. 'They'll sort it out. I once had these black things on my...'

'Not that kind of problem,' I whispered, not wanting to know about the black things. There was a momentary silence on the phone. Then:

'OK.' His voice sounded conspiratorial. 'Let's meet up.'

We met at a local pub called The Red Herring. We bought our pints and found a quiet corner. Then, leaning in, I confessed.

'Have you...' I paused. How could I talk to another man about this? Even just bringing up our sex life with anyone else felt like an infidelity. 'Have you ever had to schedule sex?'

To my surprise, Marv nodded. It was the sad nod of a man who understood the schedule. He patted the table nervously.

'Absolutely. I've been scheduling for months,' he replied. Relief overcame me. I wasn't a freak. I wasn't a freak because Marv wasn't a freak. Well, he was kind of a freak, what with the bovine thing and the inability to identify a genuine Buddhist, but in this particular instance we were both normal. Normal guys doing normal stuff. Scheduling was a straightforward, healthy part of the modern reproductive world.

'How long has you been at it?' he asked, desperate to explore our common problem. It felt good to finally meet a kindred spirit, a fellow journeyman on the road of fertility.

'About nine months,' I said.

'You dirty dog, you!' Marv stared at me with the shameful respect of two men at the gallows. Actually I have no idea what kind of look men give each other at the gallows. I imagine they don't bother much with looking. It's probably more 'Oh my god, I'm going to be hanged. From a rope. And then I'm going… hang on, is that guy eyeing me up? I swear, if he does that tomorrow I'm going to – oh, hang on…'

'You must have started just after the wedding,' Marv slapped me on the back.

Was that so unusual? Surely lots of couples threw off the shackles and went for it on their wedding night. Was it better not to rush?

Marv leaned in closer.

'The thing is,' he whispered. 'I think my wife knows.'

I looked at Marv. I was confused. Surely his wife would know about the schedule? Surely she'd be at the forefront of all scheduling activity? Martha was definitely in charge of reproductive strategy in our household, with myself in middle management and my penis taking on the role of Wally from the Dilbert cartoon. Perhaps Marv was more advanced in the art of reproductive sex, tricking his spouse into timed procreation.

'She'll kill me when she finds out,' Marv sat back, relieved, finally his secret out.

Ah, it was suddenly clear. Another woman. All the cows.

An attractive blonde walked into the bar. We both considered her. Carefully I placed my beer on the table and lowered my gaze. I felt humbled. Here I was, struggling to achieve scheduled sex with my one legitimate partner, while Marv was managing both his wife and a mistress, and he looked good on it.

'At least you haven't got her pregnant!' I laughed. But Marv didn't reply. He simply sat, his eyes following the blonde, willing her to look at him.

'Please,' I begged, clutching uncertainly at the cliffs of masculinity. 'Tell me you haven't got her pregnant?'

The blonde sat down with a group of young men. They began to laugh.

'I walk too slow,' Marv sighed, suddenly the Dalai-bloody-Lama of human reproduction. 'That's my problem. I see a herd of cows and I walk too slow.'

An hour later I arrived home to find Martha reading in bed.

'Pregnant yet?' I asked, getting undressed. Martha shook her head.

'How's your research going?'

'Brilliant,' I replied. 'Simon's congenitally deaf to the subject and Marv the Wonder Willy wants me to go on holiday and have sex with an old cow.'

'Won't be the first time for that man,' Martha tutted. I wasn't so sure – I now thought he might actually have a thing for mammals. I positioned myself on the edge of the bed.

'What about you? Anything new?' I nodded at the how-to-get-pregnant books rapidly multiplying on her bedside table.

Martha threw me a magazine. It called itself *Kitchen and Bathroom*. I took it cautiously, wondering what this had to do with baby-making. I noted that some of the pages had been tagged – Martha likes tagging things of interest to her: books, scripts, people. I once woke up with a tag on my big toe. She still won't explain that one.

I flipped to the first tag. It was a double-page advertisement featuring a beautiful woman in an evening dress. She was leaning seductively over a toilet. It was clear from her face that the toilet was turning her on and that, if I had a toilet like this, I too could invite this woman home from whatever opera she'd just attended for a night of wild, passionate toilet sex.

I visualised our own toilet. The plastic seat. The peeling paint. The cracked tile. The mountain of toilet rolls, because the one thing that could never happen in the Cossey household was a shortage of loo paper. Martha bit her nails when we got below a dozen and wasn't really comfortable with anything under thirty.

I flipped to the next tag. This time the woman was in a shower, the photo capturing the exact moment of orgasm. One tag later, she was sitting, post-coital, with her kids in the kitchen. Pages and pages were filled with women lounging by toilets, then in ecstasy as powerful nozzles pumped steamy liquid over them, and then fully dressed, opening ovens, serving home-made cakes to their beautiful children.

'We should get a new bathroom,' Martha said.

'What for?' I shrugged. How would buying a pornographic toilet help our current predicament? We needed a baby, not the orgasmatron shower head.

'Because I want one,' Martha muttered, but dropped the subject.

Another month passed and we still weren't pregnant. I was flummoxed. I had gone from one extreme to the other: for decades I had feared the unstoppable virility of my loins but it was becoming increasingly clear I had been worried about nothing.

I blame this mistaken belief on my first ever sexual experience. The one that earned me the nickname 'Two-condom Cossey'.

It was a hot, stormy evening. My parents had disappeared somewhere, and First Girlfriend had arrived for a 'study date'. Putting on a TDK SA60 cassette of early Kenny G, I lit a scented candle and ushered her into my single bed. This was the big moment, the rite of passage, the union of two bodies. Finally Mark Richard Cossey was to become a man.

Then First Girlfriend presented me with not one, but two condoms.

'You're on the pill,' I objected. I'd assumed that had removed the possibility of plastic. I didn't want plastic coming between us. No man in the universe wants plastic. Plasticman, a lesser-known superhero yet to get his own movie franchise, wouldn't wear plastic.

'And he's made of plastic,' I pleaded with First Girlfriend. Just think of the risks men take – syphilis, children – all so they don't have to wear a condom.

But like Thatcher, First Girlfriend was not for turning, or doing anything at all, until my penis was 'doubled up'. In desperation, I began to apply the condoms over my unenthusiastic member. Matters weren't helped by inexperience – I applied them the wrong way, denying myself the benefit of lubrication. I let too much air into that little bit at the end.

'You need to deflate that,' First Girlfriend said. 'It might explode inside me.'

Chance would be a fine thing. It is a benediction I still have a penis at all after that night, and nothing short of a miracle we managed to have sex successfully.

'At least we don't have to worry about a baby,' she said afterwards, studying both condoms for breakages.

First Girlfriend had left me with the conviction that pregnancy was an inevitable curse. Thanks to Two-condom Cossey I believed that a man's sperm could impregnate across space, time, alternative universes and the species barrier. Human jism was a fertility missile to be feared by all biological matter.

Now this belief lay in tatters. Getting anyone pregnant had gone from an inevitable curse to an unobtainable wish.

Over the following months scheduled sex lost its tenuous association with reality. We would, for example, try having lots of sex around ovulation. Then we'd try only having sex once, allowing my sperm to 'build up' for weeks before. We tried sex at random times, based on the theory that a watched pot never boils and that we might be able to 'sneak up' on Martha's ovaries. When that terrific idea failed we tried having sex at unusual times.

'Why are we doing this?' I asked at 3 a.m. on a Tuesday, but I don't think Martha knew.

The idea of role play came about. To spice things up. At first we were both for it, but Martha got annoyed when I tried to make her dress up as a Wood Elf.

'This isn't what I meant,' she said, waving her hands at the little green elven miniskirt. 'And put those dice away.'

I suggested bunny outfits. Then it was agreed that maybe role play wasn't for us. Did we want our firstborn conceived to the grunt of a half-orc barbarian or a strange man dressed up as Bugs Bunny?

Then, during this time of troubled sexual union, a year passed. In a few short weeks we would reach the first anniversary of both our marriage and the beginning of our quest for a baby. There were two pressing needs: get my wife pregnant and buy an anniversary present.

The traditional gift for year number one is paper. Paper. That's what you give your expectant wife when she wakes up, looks at you all doe-eyed, still feeling the romantic afterglow of those solemn vows. She waits for you to hand her a token, a sign that all is just as it was when you first uttered the words 'I do'.

'What's this?'
'It's paper! Happy anniversary!'

'It's toilet paper.'

'It's traditional. You love toilet paper.'

'It's more of a fear but…'

There was only one anniversary present that we truly wanted, and three days before we felt lucky. What a great story it would be, our firstborn conceived just in time to celebrate a year of married bliss. I rubbed my hands as I waited outside our unsexy, utilitarian toilet.

'I'm getting a restraining order if you don't move away from the door!' Martha shouted. I retreated into the living room. A few minutes later she came and sat down next to me. She lowered her head.

'Negative?'

'Negative,' she nodded.

I put my arm around her and we sat there, silent for a moment, marking the occasion. A year in and still no sign of young Indiana.

'We're not calling it Indiana,' Martha sniffed.

To make matters worse we were, once again, invited to the Morgans. I was for not going. I was for cutting the Morgans out of our lives permanently. No good was ever going to come from the Morgans.

'Leave them alone,' Martha said. 'What have they ever done to you?'

Got pregnant for starters, I thought, but said nothing and off we went, with flowers and good intentions, dragging the green gremlin behind us. We knocked on the door, promised each other that we would be kind and enthusiastic and generous. We sat at their table, ate something that may or may not have been alive once and stared into their kind, smiling faces.

'Do you want to see the scan?' Sarah clapped her hands.

'Oh they don't want to see that,' Steve shook his head.

'We'd love to,' nodded Martha, giving me a look indicating that we needed to fake our way through loving the scan.

I had no idea how to react to the weird, blurry photo in front of me. It didn't seem to represent anything at all. It was only later I realised how important that strange, black and white Polaroid of a woman's innards was.

'Wow,' I said, rotating the picture in an attempt to make sense of it, but there was nothing human growing inside Sarah.

'It looks so tiny,' Martha said, a smile pasted onto her face. Steve and Sarah continued to beam intensely.

'Does it?' Sarah clapped.

'Or?' Steve leaned forward.

'Do they?' Sarah laughed. Steve raised his eyes as if to say 'What have we done?'

It took a moment. We all sat still, the scan resting on the table.

'Twins?' Martha asked, the smile fading.

'Twins!' the Morgans chorused. 'We're having twins.'

Martha and I remained silent for a moment longer to celebrate both the Morgans' gain and the demise of our own self-respect. Then Martha left the table. We heard her go up the stairs, pause, and then open the bathroom door.

'Bugger,' we heard her say.

The door shut. Sarah looked at me.

'We've had the bathroom done.'

'Oh,' I said.

'You know, before the babies come. I think it's the nesting instinct.'

'Oh,' I continued to nod, everything clear. A state-of-the-art toilet flushed and Martha returned to the table. She smiled at our hosts. Her face was flushed, but not in the way of the women of *Kitchen and Bathroom*.

'So,' Sarah said after a moment. 'How are you both?'

Forty-eight hours later we stood on the Millennium Bridge, looking into the London night. It was our anniversary. We were dressed to the smart-casual nines, ready to celebrate our marriage.

'It's like a competition,' I said.

'A race,' Martha agreed.

We thought about the race and our position in it.

'I've never been pregnant,' Martha said.

I nodded. I tried to convince myself that there was no reason to worry. We were still well within the bounds of normality. Any month now, we could be laughing at our silly irrational fears, and asking for our money back on twenty-three ovulation kits.

That's what I had told Martha, and that's what I told myself.

That's not what I believed. What I believed, as the tourist boats floated underneath us, was everything the Internet, newspapers, TV, and my instincts were telling me. Because at twelve months everything started to scream at me: YOU'RE INFERTILE! YOU HAVE NO SPERM! YOUR TESTICLES ARE DECORATIVE APPENDAGES! Twelve months in and I had come to rue each time a dejected Martha returned from the toilet with evidence of the latest no-show of baby number one.

Twelve months and frustration was building up in the Cossey household. Martha slipped her arm around my waist. A chill wind pushed against us.

'I've tried the pants,' I cried out to the Thames. 'You've tried ovulating – whatever that is.'

Martha nodded.

'We've done the tests, the cold baths, The Calendar. We gave up drinking!'

She nodded again.

'What's left?'

Martha stared directly at me.

'A doctor,' she said. 'We need to see a doctor.'

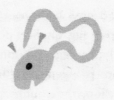

Chapter 4

Veni, Vidi, Fini

A doctor?

I don't like doctors. Bad news, delivered slow – that's the bread and butter of the doctor. Plus there's the kerfuffle: blood tests, scans, objects being stuck up places where objects shouldn't be, the excessive use of the word 'rectum'. It's not on.

Best to avoid the whole thing: lumps, wounds, a coppery taste in the mouth – in my opinion ignorance is not *a* valid form of medical treatment, it's *the* only one.

Yet now Martha was determined to get the medical profession involved. It had been two days since our anniversary and I had spent them digging my heels firmly into our laminated wooden floor, crossing my arms, and looking anywhere but into her eyes.

No one was fiddling around with my reproductive equipment.

'We're not going to any doctor,' I said.

'We are,' Martha countered, and she knew what she was talking about. She was already a walking Wikipedia of potential reproductive ills. Almost everything that could prevent pregnancy had now been memorised: endometriosis, polycystic ovaries, poor egg quality, poor sperm quality, egg hates sperm, sperm hates egg, too much sex, too little sex, varicoceles, ovulation problems, tight underwear (noted), nuclear fallout, pollution, the countryside, peanuts, fluoride, your genetic make-up, and the lambing season.

Or maybe God just hated us.

I, on the other hand, hadn't a clue. I had no idea why Martha wasn't pregnant. The mere mention of getting help conjured up terrifying images. I saw a future of numerous questions, tests, and the intensive examination of my bits. Long discussions about the state of my sex life.

Testicular massages.

Suddenly I was in an infertility IMAX cinema, witnessing my poor member being examined in 3D by giggling female medical students. Elsewhere Martha was strapped to a metal table, being poked and prodded by endless specialists, all searching for any signs of life down below. Somewhere, in the background, a string quartet was playing creepy music.

These visions came from my limited knowledge of reproductive medicine, which was based on the following: panda bears and Scully from *The X-Files*. In truth, I'm not that sure what happened to Scully, but at least she got a baby.

'Exactly,' said Martha. 'She went to a hospital and got pregnant.'

'Conception could have happened in a spaceship.'

'All right,' Martha lowered her voice. 'Can we at least accept that at some stage Scully got medical help for her fertility issues, even if it was because of intergalactic sex?'

This was the problem. Martha is smarter than me, so that even with my hazy knowledge of nineties science fiction, I was finding it difficult to argue my point. The point being that we were never, in this universe or any number of parallel ones, going to see a doctor.

She had left me with no choice: it was time to unleash the 'it'll be fine' defence.

'It'll be fine,' I said, kicking off with the classic opening.

'Oh Christ,' Martha's head hung low.

'Remember,' I began, and then paused, waiting for my brain to remember something useful. As usual it failed to do so.

'Remember...' I repeated.

'Yes?' Martha took a deep breath. Then it came to me.

'... that friend of mine – whatshisname – the one with hepatitis?'

'What's your point?'

'That turned out fine, didn't it?'

'His liver failed.'

'Really?' Typical of whatshisname. Such a lightweight. 'I thought he was fine.'

'No.'

'Still, I'm sure we'll be fine,' I finished, crossing my legs.

It is true that most instances of me saying 'it'll be fine' have ended without this being the case. I had a toothache for two years before I accepted it wouldn't be fine. That cost me fifteen hundred pounds. Then my retina detached on holiday. It took a week of walking into walls before I grudgingly agreed it wasn't going to fix itself.

'Why didn't you come in earlier?' the consultant asked.

'I thought it was fine.'

'We get a lot of that,' he sighed.

This time, with the future of our firstborn at stake, 'fine' wasn't going to cut it. I should have realised this earlier but, like men throughout the ages, I had to go through the five stages of fine: it'll be fine, it'll be fine, it'll be fine, it'll be fine, and why didn't anyone tell me it wasn't going to be fine?

Chamberlain, Poland, boy bands put together by Louis Walsh – since civilisation began, men have always thought things were going to turn out fine. After Caesar had crossed the Rubicon crying *Veni, Vidi, Fini* (I came, I saw, it'll be fine), he was shocked to feel a sharpish sensation in the lower lumbar.

'Gee, Brutus, I didn't think you were literally going to stab me in the back,' he cried.

Brutus, guilt-ridden by his dirty deed, shot a look at Cassius. 'This is going to be fine, isn't it?'

'Oh yeah, it'll be absolutely fine,' Cassius replied, wiping the blood from his toga.

As Martha and I continued to argue vis-à-vis the fineness of it all, our metaphorical fertility horizon began to darken. This was pointed out to us by The Gremlin, who now seemed to have developed some kind of rash. Honestly, he needed to see a doctor.

We studied the dark skies approaching our imminent future. What was about to hit us?

'Locusts?' I suggested.

'Babies,' Martha shuddered. 'It's the baby swarm.'

The swarm hit hard. A year ago, the existence of babies had been pure hypothesis. We knew they were out there somewhere, but they went to different parties, restaurants, nightclubs and so forth. They didn't walk on the same street – babies belonged to another country. One of those places you hear about on the news like Belarus or Panama. They exist but you're not planning a beach holiday there soon.

Now the babies were no longer on their way; they had landed and got through immigration. As Martha and I argued about medically assisted offspring, the world began to swell with everybody else's. Sinister, crying, struggling little babies.

Everywhere we went there were babies. Babies soiling nappies, babies sleeping, babies puking. Fourteen months in, I encountered our French neighbour coming up the stairs.

She looked tired and haggard. What could be the cause of her ennui? Merlot? Post-modernism?

'This is Françoise,' she smiled wearily, offering up a crazy-looking mummified thing wrapped in a cotton shawl.

'A good-looking lad,' I said. It wasn't. To be honest, it looked like it was from Mordor. Or Rodrom as they probably call it in France with their perverse, back-to-front spelling ways.

'She. It is a *girl*,' she huffed, disappearing into her flat. I sighed. That was the baby we could hear sometimes. A French baby.

Call me an anti-Francophile freedom-loving hero of Anglo-Saxon liberalism and decency if you like, but French babies are the worst. They cry in French, grow up to be French and then start telling you how good the French are. Really? Open your shops on a Monday then. Win a land war. Stop missing the whole German army invading from the north and stop calling two islands and an atoll an empire. No one even knows what an atoll is.

At least British babies grow up to tell you how rubbish their country is and how they're not British but Welsh/Scottish/a Londoner/not from around here anyway.

That night the French baby began to wail in earnest. It's always tricky, living next to something whose *raison d'être* is howling, but try having scheduled sex, sober, with that and a sleep-deprived Parisian shouting '*merde*' and see how you get on. The French factor led to increased pressure from Martha for us to get outside help.

'Look,' I said, frustrated that she couldn't see how fine everything was. 'If I say it's going to be fine, it is going to be fine.'

'No,' she replied, clenching her fists in frustration. 'You use the word "fine" as a replacement for the whole English language. You saying it's fine is like saying the universe will or will not continue.'

'You're just generalising.' I waved a finger at her. Martha was always generalising. It was a fault in her personality.

'I'm not generalising. I specifically, in a very un-general way, without any ambiguity whatsoever, want to go to see a doctor. What is wrong with going to see a doctor?'

My gaze fell.

'I don't...' I held my breath. I didn't want the words to come out, but they did. 'I don't want to know. I just don't want to know.'

Martha looked at me. Her face softened. Her hand went to my cheek.

'Please, Roo,' she said, and there was something in her voice. I couldn't place it for a moment, because I had never heard her express it before. But there it was: a strained note at the end of her sentence.

The faintest hint of desperation.

I called my sister. Emily lived over ten thousand miles away in a small country town in Australia called Queanbeyan. It's the home of George Lazenby, who played James Bond in the seventies and we had always been close. Not me and George, you understand, me and my sister.

Actually that's not true. As children, we were sworn enemies. Our house was like Bosnia in the nineties. I once nailed all her soft toys to her bedroom wall, except her favourite pink bunny, which I hung from the ceiling light. Then I waited and listened with a sort of horrified ecstasy to her high-pitched scream as she was confronted by the massacre.

To those toys I was Slobodan Milosevic. I should've been done for war crimes or at least had my pocket money docked, but instead Emily forgave me, which was not bad at all for an eight-year-old.

'We're thinking about going to a doctor,' I confessed.

In the background I could her daughter crying for something.

'Grant,' she shouted away from the phone. 'Can you sort Abbey out?'

Abbey was momentarily silenced and my sister returned to the phone.

'You want an honest answer?'

'Mmmm,' I wasn't sure.

'I think it's all right. Honestly, lots of people have problems these days.'

'Really?'

'Uh-huh.'

There was another pause. Then Emily said:

'There's something else I've got to tell you. I'm pregnant.'

There was no Slobodan left in me. I was only happy for her. She was one person I could never begrudge anything.

A day later I gave in. Martha and I sat in a cafe, laughing at people ordering soya milk lattes. It's funny because soya milk tastes like cardboard. Later I discovered it's also funny because I read somewhere soya has enough oestrogen to affect a woman's menstrual cycle and damage the quality of men's sperm. Soya is nature's way of neutering hippies and those people who get wooden boxes of random vegetables delivered to their door.

'Look, the vegetable box has arrived!'

'Oh great, I'll pop the tofu in the oven.'

'Here's a mouldy cabbage, here's a gourd, and is this a mushroom?'

'All right,' I said, as another pram with parents attached strolled in to the cafe. 'We'll go to the doctor. Just to – you know.' I paused. 'Make sure it's fine.'

Martha nodded. She rubbed my back and then moved her hand to my shoulder and pulled me towards her. Her husband might be slow, but he got there in the end.

Two days later, we sat opposite our GP. It's an odd thing, going to the doctor. You go in with a predetermined attitude, an idea of what you want and how you're going to get it. Some people like to play up their symptoms. It's all, 'Oooh, Doctor, it's painful,' and 'I don't think it's the right shape anymore,' and so on. Personally, I find this over-egging a pathetic, time-wasting, moral weakness of character, depriving others of much-needed medical resources.

My tactic involved downplaying everything. I liked to deny the doctor any useful information whatsoever. They're the experts, let them work it out. If they looked young and inexperienced I might give a little clue like, 'It's not that bad,' or 'I'm sure it'll grow back,' and so on, but otherwise they were on their own. I don't know a GP in the land who doesn't respect the patient who kicks off the conversation with the immortal words:

'It's probably nothing...'

It is true that the occasional doctor gets annoyed at this sort of noble, stoic behaviour.

'So what do you think is wrong?'

'Probably nothing.'

'And when did this nothing start?'

'Never.'

'You know we only have ten minutes...'

They're also trained not to judge their patients. Once my face swelled up to the extent where I was a dead ringer for the Elephant Man. The high-pitched screams each time Martha was confronted by her balloon-faced partner made me realise I needed help and soon enough I was sitting in front of my GP, who took one look at me, blew out some air and leaned away.

'So,' he said. 'What seems to be the problem, Mr Merrick?'

'What?'

'I said what seems to be the problem, Mr Cossey?'

'Well it's probably nothing but I look like the Elephant Man.'

The GP stared blankly at my face.

'Is that normal?'

Beat.

'Do you think it's normal?'

We skipped into our doctor's room, beaming with false happiness, trying to give the impression of two virile, sex-mad bunnies who are up for anything. Sitting down, I slouched a little so he could get a good view of the exceptionally loose pants hanging out from the top of my jeans.

'Fertility problems?' he asked.

He was a nice man, our GP, a tall cockney German. I don't know how that happened. His Teutonic accent banged alongside an East End attitude and somehow it was all very comforting. He encouraged us to tell him everything. We went into detail. Perhaps too much detail. Martha told him how she had missed a period at sixteen and I described the ovulation kits and the scheduled sex and my lost *Wisden*.

'I do not need to know about the cricket,' he said, stopping me mid flow.

'Right,' I nodded. Fair enough.

'And those tests to tell you when you're ovulating?'

The nod again.

'Useless.'

'What?'

'They don't work. Once you know you're ovulating, which you have clearly proven beyond doubt, they do not increase your chances of pregnancy.'

'But they work, though?' Martha pleaded. 'The chemist said...'

'Ja, ja, they work technically. But they don't work statistically, you see?'

I had no idea what he was talking about but Martha lowered her head, crestfallen. The tests had been at the top of her infertility arsenal. Sensing harm done, the GP softened his voice.

'You've been trying about a year, ja?'

We nodded.

'And you, you know, have the sex? A few times a week?'

We continued nodding. He knew us too well.

'Not too close together?'

Us or the sex?

'What you need to do is not panic, and keep having the sex. No too much of the sex, not too little. Ja?'

Scientific stuff. Like our other doctor, the Internet, he assured us that most people who failed to get pregnant in their first year conceived naturally in their second. If we were still having problems at the two-year point, then we could look at some treatment.

And that was that. I confess my feelings were mixed: on the one hand I was relieved – no one in the medical world was going to be cupping my scrotal sack in their palms just yet. I had another year for my sperm to lift its game and get Martha pregnant.

On the other hand it did mean another year of dancing to the tune of The Sex Calendar on the fridge door. That, I wasn't so thrilled about. Neither was Martha – her nesting instinct was going into overdrive and she was already firmly convinced that the God of Hubris had destined her to a life of childlessness.

After the visit to the doctor I began to notice other subtle changes in my wife's behaviour. Little things, like the television, which used to be set to *Breakfast* first thing in the morning, was now left off. Now we listened to the posh folk on Radio 4 discussing inequality with south London rap artists.

'What happened to the telly?' I asked.

'It's out to get us,' Martha said.

Poor little woman, I thought. Poor, dear little Roo. The stress of it all had finally gotten too much for her.

'How is it out to get us?' I asked gently.

'It just is.'

I took her over and sat her on the sofa. I picked up the remote control and waited for the TV to boot up.

'Roo,' I said. 'The TV is not out to...'

'... a new study suggests that men soaking in the bath reduces sperm count by 491 per cent...' the presenter said. She went on to explain that men who didn't bath had a significantly better sperm count than those who did. An expert in sperm then predicted that by next June there would be not be a single human sperm in the world anywhere and that the human race was on the verge of dying out and...

I turned the TV off.

'OK,' I agreed. 'It's out to get us.'

Morning TV wasn't the only one. The newspapers were full of stories about fertility rates dropping because of adequate hot water supplies or women waiting until they're ready to have a baby. The tabloids especially seemed to believe that anyone who hadn't started pumping out kids by eighteen had betrayed the human race.

I did wonder how they found these things out. What kind of tests were performed? Was there a secret lab in Switzerland next to the Large Hadron Collider, full of men masturbating in differently heated baths? Women in black leather body suits, whipping laggards who weren't 'productive enough'.

'You need help,' Martha said, making burgers for dinner.

Then she suggested that maybe we should both talk to someone. About feelings. I was against the idea. I am, in general, against talking to people. Talking is overrated. Israel and the Palestinians never stop going on at each other and look where it's got them.

When I was younger I was sent to a psychiatrist to 'talk', possibly about the soft-toy incident. Anyway, the man was a right nutter. He appeared to have only two counselling techniques: forcing his patients to read *The Alexandria Quartet* by Lawrence Durrell and getting them to imagine worst-case scenarios. Why would imagining things being worse make you feel better? There you were, depressed, the full futility of life pressed up against you, having just discovered that Durrell had also penned a quintet, and you were expected to imagine being diagnosed with a brain tumour. What did he expect people to do? Cheer up?

'So how's that Durrell going for you?' he would ask at the beginning of each session.

'It's boring, depressing, wallowing crap.'

'I see.' He would write something on his notepad. 'And did you imagine some worst-case scenarios?'

'I tried but, to be honest, reading a non-linear series of novels and then talking to you about them is pretty much my personal Armageddon...'

I suppose it was successful in the sense that I haven't taken my own life, so I suggested to Martha that we might try and imagine our own worst-case scenario: a childless future.

'Can't we just get some professional help?' she begged.

We sat down and began to imagine our childless future. We tried hard to think what would be different, how we might feel and so on, but it was the oddest thing: it didn't feel any different at all. Suddenly we realised we were already childless. We had no children. We were not part of the swarm. We didn't even have a goldfish due to the restrictions on our lease. The future was just like now, but Radio 2 would probably start to feel cool and maybe tight perms would come back into fashion.

'I'm scared,' said Martha.

'Of curlers?'

'That we might only have each other?'

I considered the prospect. There had always been a part of me that would be happy with this outcome. I imagined Martha and I getting old together, I imagined her making cups of tea and me claiming to be translating Plato in the loft but actually playing SimCity. Actually that's still a lie; I would be playing online Dungeons & Dragons as a wizard. And what a wizard I would be!

Anyway, I had always felt guilty about this little dream, as though I was willing our theoretical children away.

Now I realised that I had completely misunderstood my own fantasy-role-playing future. This imaginary universe was based on the solid ground that somewhere, nearby, were our children. Children underfoot interrupting Martha's specific method for tea-brewing. Children ringing us up needing money for 'books' at university. Children married to someone with parents who weren't quite right in the head.

It was suddenly clear that without kids, everything about our future would collapse. There would be no loft, no tea, no...

... no Martha?

'OK,' I said, suddenly frightened. 'This is a stupid game.'

Martha nodded. Then the French baby started crying again and then, moments later, there was a knock at the door. I went to answer it.

Standing there was Agnes, the aging West Country socialite from downstairs, dressed in a spotless white bathrobe and velvet slippers. I say socialite because she had a tendency to segue into name-dropping at the first opportunity, though they were never names anyone had heard of. Still, when sober, she was friendly enough.

'The baby,' she slurred, staring nowhere with unfocused fury. 'Is it yours?'

Agnes was not sober. I shook my head and pointed at the door opposite.

'Little beast,' she spat bitterly. 'We're lucky – lucky that we don't have these little bastards. Complete waste of time.'

Then she turned from me, tensed her shoulders, and prepared to do battle with the French mother. I closed the door and looked at Martha.

'I'm scared,' Martha grimaced.

That night, we lay in bed, listening to the Parisians surrendering the last of their self-respect. They were now openly begging their baby to stop screaming. That having failed, they began to scream back at it, then at each other, then it ceased to become clear who was screaming at whom, and soon enough Agnes joined in from the corridor, until the noise morphed into one hellish scream montage, except that usually in a montage you get a sense of time passing.

Then came the text on Martha's phone. She picked it up, opened the message, and then threw it against the wall.

TRYING

I retrieved the phone and looked at the message.

'Girl and boy, born 1812 and 1816, both happy and healthy. The Morgans.'

I turned around. Martha was on the computer, searching the Internet.

'Baby assassin?' I asked.

'Private clinic,' she replied.

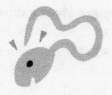

Chapter 5

Money, Irony and Lies

The receptionist smiled at us and I regretted wearing my two-year-old trainers. We had arrived at the private clinic. The waiting rooms were a delight; the chairs had arms and padded seats and the floor wasn't cheap lino, and the customers, or clients, or whatever we were called, were all smartly dressed and respectable-looking.

In an instant we were ushered into a spacious, sunlit consultation room. More comfortable seating was provided. Someone brought us coffee. A Rolex-clad consultant entered, greeting us with a perfect, multimillionaire smile. He had clearly done well out of the infertile, which was unsurprising considering the costs. Martha had shown me the price list the previous evening.

'Bejeezus,' I had cried, or words to that effect, spitting lamb vindaloo over our Xthorp rug. £5,000. For a round of IVF. £5,000 to have a bloody baby.

'It's not a guarantee.' Back in the sunny room the consultant outlined the process to us. 'Assuming nothing is medically wrong, you've probably got about a thirty per cent chance per cycle of IVF.'

Thirty per cent? £5,000 for less than a one-in-three chance of getting pregnant?

'They're good odds,' he smiled. 'We're one of the best clinics in the country.'

It's not a guarantee. Where were we going to get £5,000 on a regular basis from?

'It's a drop in the ocean,' Martha said. 'When you think how much it costs to raise a child.'

'I don't want to know!' I covered my ears.

'Two hundred thousand,' she smiled.

'What?' This wasn't a rhetorical 'what'. I actually had covered my ears and couldn't hear what she was saying. So Martha wrote it on a Post-it note and showed me.

TWO HUNDRED THOUSAND POUNDS, it said.

I closed my eyes, but it was too late. Martha stuck the note on my forehead. Two hundred thousand pounds for each child.

The three of us – the consultant, Martha and I – sat silently for a moment, sipping our coffee. Suddenly, a hologram of the Skeletors, standing on that rooftop, appeared on the table.

'Do you actually want this? Do you?'

Then it was gone.

'What if there is something wrong?' Martha asked.

The consultant fiddled with the bevel on his watch and looked away.

'That depends,' he said, 'on what's up and how bad it is.'

His smile returned. He told us to go home and think it through. *Come back when you're desperate,* he seemed to be saying. *Then you'll pay me whatever I ask.*

We went home. It was not obvious how we could fund a lengthy fertility campaign. Assuming there was nothing wrong with us, and assuming it took three attempts to conceive, it was, with egg storage and the other extras, going to cost us north of twenty thousand pounds.

'Ironic,' noted Martha, looking at our four walls.

It was. Twenty thousand was the sum total of our wealth until about six months ago when we had used every last penny to buy our flat. A flat big enough to have a baby in.

A baby we now couldn't afford.

Could we ask our parents for help? It was not clear. My mother had passed away many years ago. My father was an academic mathematician. This did not make him a man of the world. He asked strangers to mind his bags at airports. He almost wore a tracksuit to meet the Governor General of Australia. It had been nearly a quarter of a century since our last discussion on the subject of reproduction and that had concerned birth control.

'Never used it,' he said, clashing the gears on his old VW Combi.

'What, never?'

'Nope.'

'What about Mum?'

'Had kids.'

'And then?'

'Had an operation.'

If ever I didn't want to know something, it was who had the operation.

'It was your mother.'

'What about other girlfriends?' It was the swinging sixties after all.

'Weren't any.'

Martha's parents were a better bet, but even there we baulked. They were very involved with their daughter, just not always in a useful way. For example, in the first flat where we first began 'trying', Martha's father could see into our bedroom from their flat across the road. Sometimes he would ring up in the afternoon.

'Why are the curtains closed?'

'Dad!'

'Is Mark ill?'

'No...'

'Are you ill?'

'Dad!'

We moved.

They didn't want to interfere. They had always encouraged Martha to be independent but as time passed they did become curious about the potential for grandchildren. It came up in subtle, little ways.

'You don't want to worry about it,' Martha's mum would say, apropos of nothing.

'About what?'

'Nothing. That's what I'm saying. Don't worry about anything. It doesn't help worrying.'

'It doesn't help worrying about nothing?'

'That's what I'm saying.'

'We're not worried!'

But we were. We were worried enough to talk about selling the flat. About trying to get a loan despite the large mortgage. Extending the overdraft, upping the credit limit on the Barclaycard.

Scratch lotto.

Yet something held me back. I thought it was the money. I couldn't bring myself to spend cash on what was supposed to be the free part of the whole thing. Why should I pay to find out how badly damaged our reproductive organs were? Why did I have to pay for some elaborate medical procedure with a lousy statistical outcome?

Why should I pay for a baby?

I prepared myself for a showdown with Martha. I was sure she wanted to get started, to spare no expense: she would want to sell the flat, to be in hock to every bank in the country, she would want us to become drug mules or prostitutes. She was a formidable foe, so I picked our traditional time for an argument: Saturday morning.

It's always best to argue on a Saturday. Then you can really give it some space. Allow the dispute the full spectrum of behaviour on an unbroken timeline: sulking, shouting, sarcasm, throwing things, leaving, coming back, packing, leaving again – this time for good – standing in the rain, returning, cup of tea, having a sub-argument about who should actually do the leaving, threatening to leave if the other doesn't, both leaving together – until finally, having forgotten what the original fight was about, resolving everything with make-up sex at around 11.20 p.m. on Sunday.

Saturday mornings. The time for a fight.

'I don't think we should do it,' I said at 9.01 a.m., flicking on the kettle switch.

Martha held a tea bag over my mug.

'Why?' she asked.

'Money.'

Martha didn't move. I closed my eyes. Something bad was coming. This was going to be the granddaddy of all Cossey arguments. This was going to…

'I agree,' she said. The tea bag fell into the mug. The kettle boiled.

I looked up at the clock. 9.04.

'O-K,' I said. I felt no relief. For starters, what were we going to do for the next forty-eight hours? Also, something wrong had happened, a disturbance in the Cossey force, an unknown evil forestalled but not faced.

We spent six months tinkering around the edges. We talked less and less about getting pregnant and spent more time with our single friends. The Gremlin went with Marv to Vietnam to find himself and the testing kits disappeared.

'People conceived before those tests,' Martha shrugged.

We bought a jigsaw.

'I'm going to do it ironically,' I made it clear, surveying the selection of jigsaws at John Lewis, one of which we were going to assemble in our ironic flat. I was amazed at how bad the pictures were.

'This is a picture of deer,' I said. 'In a woodland.'

Martha browsed silently.

'And here,' I continued, 'is a train. On a mountain.'

'What do you want on a jigsaw?' Martha asked. 'Nudity?'

I knew a man who started a business in pornographic jigsaws. It was not a success. The market for people who wanted to delay gratification to that extent turned out to be exactly two, and it's possible his mum was just being nice.

'Bruce Willis,' I replied. 'Jumping onto a plane. From a truck.'

'Did that happen?' Martha picked up a box with the Battle of Waterloo on it.

It did. That's the problem when you make an action film whose central threat is a computer virus. Nothing happens and you end up doing something stupid.

'I'm going to jump onto a Harrier Jet?'

'It's more a leap and then a fall.'

'Wouldn't my character just reboot the computer or something?'

'Bruce...'

'It just feels like we're jumping the shark here.'

'No one's jumping a shark. You're leaping onto a jet. From a truck.'

In the end we chose a one-thousand-piece ruined Welsh castle with a flock of birds flying over it. Over the next few days I began to realise you didn't 'play' a jigsaw. You 'start' a jigsaw. Then you 'finish' it. A jigsaw is so dull that there is no verb to describe the process of jigsawing. It is a meaningless and pointless activity and, on top of that, difficult. All those pieces. Which have to fit together. It was this combination of dull, aching difficulty that drove us into the arms of the scheduled sex which we were pretending not to have.

Five days of jigsaw-puzzling later, I noticed Martha had begun to scribble numbers down on a pad.

'What,' I asked. 'Is this?'

'I'm keeping score.'

'What?'

'I'm keeping score of how many pieces I get.'

'But you don't know how many pieces I've got,' I snapped.

'I'll minus my number off the finished puzzle and then we'll know who won.'

'You can't win at jigsaw!' I left the room.

Only my wife would turn a jigsaw into a competitive sport. I looked at the scorecard. She had now placed 436 pieces. I looked at the bits of attached cardboard in front of me. It was not, in any sense, near finished.

'This isn't ironic,' I objected, but it was too late. Soon we were furiously competing to recreate the photo of the castle. Our relationship became strained when Martha accused me of hiding pieces (they were just resting in my bag) and three days later it was over. I learned two lessons: firstly, Martha was better at jigsaws.

The second was triggered by a chance encounter with Mrs Skeletor. She had recently joined the BBC, and one warm August day I walked past her sitting on a bench outside, talking into her phone. I was about ten feet away when I overheard the conversation.

'It's not about that.' Her voice shook. 'It's the house. It's more efficient if we do it this way...'

Her grey, thin face turned to me, her gaze met mine. I expected a hollowed-out stare, but her eyes, though bloodshot, still had warmth about them. She gave me a faint smile as though apologising for something. Then she turned away and continued to talk into her phone.

Sorry for what? I wondered.

I walked on. Then it hit me. Something evil wasn't coming. We had avoided nothing. Evil had arrived.

IVF is not a guarantee.

Do you really want it, do you?

That night, when Martha walked in the door, she found me waiting for her on the couch. In my left hand I held a single pregnancy kit.

'Ah,' she said, scratching her chin. Without talking, I led her into the bedroom. On the bed were nineteen packets of assorted fertility-testing kits I had discovered hidden around the flat.

'Boo.' I looked at her. Martha lowered her head.

'I'm frightened,' she said.

'Of not having a baby?'

She shook her head slowly.

'Of knowing. I don't want to know either.'

There it was. The truth. We wanted a baby, but we were too scared to find out if we could have one or not.

After all, wasn't it easier to sit in our little flat, with our hidden tests and our monthly disappointments and our crazy rituals? Wasn't it better to hide away?

I was all for hiding. I was the first to suggest not knowing and sticking our heads in the sand. I was the one who said it was going to be fine. The last thing I wanted was to sit in some room and be told we were never going to have a child. To see Martha break down in tears. To take her home, the home we had bought for the baby, the baby that would now never exist. To make that first cup of tea knowing you would never have a son or daughter to call your own. That was the evil. Who could live with that?

And yet.

'Roo.' My forehead touched hers. 'Roo.'

Martha's head remained bowed.

'We're going to fight this,' I whispered. Martha looked up. What kind of fighting?

'We're going to do something wrong,' I said. 'But we're going to do it for the baby. Our baby, which we are going to have.'

I let her go. I picked up my Allan Border signed cricket bat and slapped the face of it in my palm. Then three puffins materialised on my wife. One on her head, another on her shoulder, a third nestled like a baby in her arms. They were small, these flightless birds, no taller than a wine bottle, and they stared at me with a collective expression that was so, so pitiful. They radiated a kind of sorrowful cuteness.

Then, with the blink of an eye, they were gone.

'We,' I said to Martha, 'are going back to the GP.'

Martha looked up at her husband. This is partly because I don't allow a heeled shoe in my presence, but also because I had risen in stature. We were going to conquer this thing.

'How?' Martha asked. 'We've got to wait another four months – and getting the money to go private will take...' How could I ignore the fact that, according to the NHS, we were still within the normal boundaries? How could I ignore the fact that, according to the two-tier British health system, we were too poor to get pregnant?

'We lie,' I said. I was steel. Blue steel.

'Lie?'

'Lie.'

Martha considered this option.

'And if we got caught?'

'They can't test for long-ago sex.'

'But we told them about long-ago sex.'

'We miscounted.'

I was correct: they cannot dust a woman's uterus for sperm. They cannot remove a strand of pubic hair and match its DNA with the romp we had two years ago. It was the perfect crime. Who was to say that we hadn't been at it for decades? We were invulnerable.

Our fraudulent pact agreed, we returned to the GP. Our deceit was to have the quiet confidence of Bernie Madoff and the righteousness of Nixon. The key thing, as I saw it, was to keep it simple. Whatever was thrown at us, we needed to stick to the mantra that we'd been trying for two years.

We entered the consulting room to face our destiny.

'Um,' I said. 'We've being trying for two years.'

Our GP studied us, suspicious. He looked at his screen.

'My records,' – his voice seemed more Germanic now – 'say otherwise.'

Foiled! All our hard painstaking work ruined by a freak example of accurate NHS record-keeping.

'Your records are wrong.'

'Why would our records be wrong?'

'Two years,' we bleated in unison.

Cosseys against the world. He knew the game. We wanted a baby and we wanted it born yesterday. He had budgets to protect and infertility was somewhere below a verruca on the priority list. We had the human race to continue. He had Mrs Gomez at 10.30 for a check-up on her haemorrhoids.

Like a hardened bouncer, he loosened his shoulders and turned towards his computer screen, emotionless. He began typing.

'OK,' he said. 'You're in.'

Result! I cheered silently. High fives and back slaps all round. We had told a lie and it had worked. I imagined other lies I could start telling. Sick days off work. No more overcooked food at the Morgans. I could work in banking or become a lawyer or be a courier with a two-hour delivery window. A sweet, rich future lay ahead for the new, deceitful, Cosseys!

Then Martha started to cry.

'You OK?' asked the GP.

'It's the lies,' she said. 'I can't handle the lies.'

The doctor looked at me. I wracked my brain. Martha was about to mess everything up and I had to do something. I needed a cunning plan. What was causing Martha to cry? An affair? She's having an affair? No, hang on, then I'd be crying. She'd be fine, the traitorous cow. No, no, let's say I'm having an affair. With Billie Piper. That's good, adds a little glamour. But why, given the fact that my wife had just found out I'm sleeping with a famous actress, are we still trying for a baby? To save the marriage? To…

'We're lying,' I nodded, lowering my face. The relief of a condemned man flowed through me. 'We haven't been trying for two years, we've only been at it for twenty months!'

'Nineteen and a half,' Martha sniffed.

'Nineteen and a half,' I agreed.

The doctor stared at us. It hadn't turned out well, our plan. The truth was we were never up to the job. We were the worst liars in the world. We would often confess before anyone even suggested we'd done something wrong. We would admit to things that we hadn't done, such was the fear that we might inadvertently be lying.

'You…' The doctor paused, looking at us both. The room chilled. Were we in trouble? Was the NHS fraud division coming to arrest us? 'You are terrible liars.' His voice softened. 'But maybe you will be better parents.'

He clicked the mouse of his computer a couple of times, typed in a few letters and then turned back to us.

'You're still in,' he smiled. 'Good luck.'

We smiled back. Cheats never prosper, I thought. Well, except for the fact we'd attempted to defraud the NHS and that the doctor had cheated to get us in, but let's not ruin the moment.

For some fortunate reason our health trust funded fertility treatment. Understood that committed parents-to-be were worth taking a punt on. Later, I discovered that much of the NHS tries to avoid having anything to do with fertility. I don't know why. Someone in the NHS had decided that teeth, which you need to eat, and reproduction, which you need to breed, weren't critical to the survival of humanity. Go figure.

We were lucky; we had won the postcode lottery, which in itself also seemed a little unsettling. The idea of health administrators gambling. With lives. I guess it must be a real step up if you're a bingo addict, but it's an odd image for socialised medicine.

'Do they have the lotto for other conditions?' I asked the GP.

'Oh yes,' he smiled. 'Now I'm going to send you to the South Morden.'

An alarm bell sounded in my mind.

'Isn't St William's closer?' St William's was the hospital nearest our flat. We basically lived next to Willy's.

'Yes, but your local PCT is in Morden.'

Whatever a PCT was, it didn't sound very local.

'But I can see St William's from my window.'

'You'll be going to the Morden.'

In our desperation to get started we agreed to this. We agreed to go to a hospital miles away in deepest, darkest south London rather than fight for the one next to our home.

This was a mistake. Inside my head the bells rang louder. The damned cried out my name. The people of Morden held vigils, warning us to stay away, and if I had listened we wouldn't have wasted another year in our search for a baby. If I had listened I might have been a father in my thirties.

If I had listened we never would have met The Wicked Witch of South Morden.

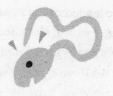

Chapter 6

The Wicked Witch of South Morden

I was showing some colleagues around the set of the TARDIS when The Wicked Witch called.

'Mr Cossey?' came the squeal of her high-pitched voice. 'You do realise your sample was due today.'

'No, it's tomorrow.'

'It's today.'

'I'm in Pontypridd.'

'Today. Before one o'clock.'

She hung up. I looked at my watch. Five past ten. I was fifteen miles out of Cardiff in a TV studio with two bearded *Doctor Who* obsessives and no transport, and in the next three hours I somehow needed to get back to London, travel across town and deliver a sample of my sperm to the South Morden hospital. When, where and how I was going to produce this sample was unclear.

I looked wistfully at the controls of the TARDIS. If only...

'One more photo?' pleaded the man with the largest acreage of facial hair. Sighing, I raised the camera. Making a family was one thing, but Doctor Who waited for no one.

Two hours later I was on a train suffering minor delays near Swindon. The train wasn't the only thing not moving. I'd already had 'a go' in the toilets, but you try masturbating into a jar for the first time on the Great Western line. Anyone who has experienced the journey from Cardiff to London will know it's just not conducive to this sort of activity. I had tried to call The Wicked Witch and beg her to postpone delivery, but she wasn't picking up.

I was in trouble and it was mostly her fault.

It had all started two weeks before, when Martha and I first arrived at the South Morden. I don't want to speak ill of the place. It was ill enough. It was the most disorganised institution I'd encountered, and I once worked in the mail room of an Australian government department that decided to rename itself DOPIE. I'm sure the good doctors and nurses did their best, but entropy had a better organisational structure than the administration of that collection of buildings which happened to have the name 'Hospital' slapped on them.

Somewhere in this strange place, off to the side in its own forgotten little corner, was the fertility clinic. And lurking inside, like that spider in *The Lord of the Rings*, was a woman: The Wicked Witch of South Morden. So named, by myself, because she was wicked and a witch, and because she needed taking out by a flying bungalow.

She had clearly misunderstood when she signed up for a career in the NHS.

'I want to do anti-natal.'

'Sure.'

'Will I be stopping people having children?'

'Actually, it's antenatal.'

'That's what I said.'

'No, it's spelled with a... oh, what the hell, just sign here. We'll dump you in fertility.'

It's hard to imagine now, but when we first arrived at the hospital Martha and I were full of something called hope. The Wicked Witch was still ten minutes or so from entering our lives and, like innocent lambs, we bounced optimistically up to the front desk, which was manned by a single security guard.

'Think, Roo.' Martha held my hand tightly. 'We might actually be getting closer to our little baby!'

She was like Dorothy having discovered the yellow brick road and I was like, well, whoever Dorothy would have ended up with after the onset of puberty. The Scarecrow? That would be an uncomfortable night. Maybe the Tin Man, but then again, there's no evidence that he was anatomically correct; and the Lion, well that would be illegal except in Germany so...

'Who's Dorothy?' Dorothy asked, before morphing back into Martha.

Manfully, I asked the guard for directions to the fertility clinic. A shadow fell over his face – it was as if I'd asked for the morgue.

'Difficult,' he said.

'Really?'

'Very difficult. I reckon you'll need someone to show you.'

It was soon clear that this someone was not him, or indeed, anyone who worked at the Morden. Finally, he did manage to scrawl some directions on the back of a pamphlet marked 'Here to help' and, following it with a yet undampened zeal, we ended up in Gastroenterology.

There Peter, a nice man, slightly nervous about his upcoming colonoscopy, showed us to a well-concealed fire door. He seemed strangely familiar with our navigational plight.

'Best of luck,' he smiled, conspiratorially pushing us back outside the hospital.

We went down a lane, past what may or may not have been an incinerator before finally arriving at a large, dirty Portakabin next to two rubbish skips. A piece of paper was taped to its door. The words 'Reproductive Medicine' were printed on it in Comic Sans, the font of the incompetent, with a little smiley face underneath.

It looked like the hospital had run out of money just as they'd reached Fertility. A bit like the finale of the second *Tomb Raider* film. You know the one: Lara Croft charges all over the world, fighting Chinese ninjas, blowing stuff up, jet packing, etc, and then she ends up in a small, badly made set, purporting to be a cave in Africa.

In front of her is a tatty IKEA *Motorp* storage unit. She looks up at the director:

'That's Pandora's box? The most powerful force in the universe?'

'Yep.'

'It's in a puddle.'

'It's like the *Raiders* film. Everything's meant to be simple, intense.'

'So it's protected by tons of ingenious traps then?'

'Not exactly, but it is quite hard to reach.'

'What?'

'You'll have to stretch.'

'I save the world by stretching?'

'Yep.'

'And when the box is opened? Then we get some kind of horrific monster, right?'

'Here's the brilliant bit. You don't.'

'I don't get any horrific monsters?'

'You don't open the box.'

'I don't?'

'You just leave it.'

'So I stretch out to the box and then decide to leave it?'

'Uh-huh.'

Pause.

'That's the end of your film?'

We went in. At first, there was a comforting sight: a waiting room full of people. Standard for the NHS, but the thing was they were all *normal*. Normal in the sense that they were like us. About the same age, limbs intact, all carrying the same look of wistful optimism that somehow medical science was going to sort out in the test tube what they couldn't in the bedroom.

Then, from behind the reception, The Wicked Witch materialised. She was a short, thin-lipped woman: who knew that underneath such a modest, mousy-haired appearance lay an evil ready to suck all that was good from our world.

At first we tried to be friendly. She couldn't find our notes. We smiled patiently. She wasn't convinced we'd come on the right day. Nor was she convinced that we hadn't. Then she became annoyed when a colleague, some kind of good munchkin who had snuck in under the radar, proved to her that we had arrived on the correct date and that our notes were in a Manila folder with Martha's name printed clearly on it.

Temporarily frustrated, The Wicked Witch instructed us to wait. There was now a lengthy line of people behind us who she needed to be unpleasant to.

I asked how long it might be until we'd see a doctor.

'We're busy.'

'Yes, I can see that but…'

'Sit down and wait.'

We sat down and waited. For a long, long time we waited. Then we waited some more.

I am not a good waiter. Martha has observed this. The thing I hate most in life is waiting. If I was on death row, I wouldn't bother with an appeal; such is my dislike of the wait. I would tell them to get it over with so we could all just move on with our lives.

'But you wouldn't move on, Mr Cossey. You'd be dead.'

'But I won't have to wait?'

'You won't have to wait.'

'Well then.'

Finally a consultant appeared from the inner sanctum of the Portakabin and called out Martha's name. Saved! In another minute we were crushed into a tiny office, the consultant flipping through our notes. He turned to Martha.

'First, you will have the tests.'

For Martha, that meant blood tests for everything up to and including HIV, an ultrasound, a good poking down there, and an X-ray. Sounded pretty horrific for her, but at least I wasn't waiting. We nodded enthusiastically, willing to take anything on. For the family. For Bob.

'We're not calling it Bob,' Martha whispered.

Then the consultant turned to me, winking at me in a two-men-who-know-what's-what kind of way.

'And for you, also the HIV test.'

'Great!' I beamed, wondering what the correct response to being offered an HIV test was. 'I mean fine. I mean that seems sensible.'

The consultant gave me a little nudge.

'Don't worry, if it's positive, we can clean up your sperm.'

Wow, I thought. I'll have HIV, which I would have probably passed onto my wife, what with all the unscheduled sex we'd been having, but at least our orphaned child won't have to worry about AIDS while being criminalised in a government orphanage. I returned his nudge to indicate how impressed I was with this advance in medical science. He raised a hand.

'Please. We clean up all sorts of stuff these days. Hepatitis, HIV, it's all good.'

I nodded. It was impressive stuff, but I didn't fancy either condition. My auto immune system was already prone to man flu and my liver had been through enough, what with the now semi-permanent reduction in alcohol and processed red meat.

'... and of course, we will need the sample.'

The sample. We all knew what that meant. Martha and I chuckled, the doctor chuckled, all very amusing. The sample.

'And then you'll be able to tell us what's wrong?' Martha asked.

The consultant leaned back in his chair, opened his hands, and looked towards the ceiling as if appealing to the heavens.

'Sometimes,' he said wistfully. 'Sometimes we can see, sometimes we just don't know. It's about fifty-fifty.' Fifty-fifty? Only a fifty per cent chance of diagnosing the problem, let alone fixing it? What had medicine been up to on the fertility front?

'It's the mystery of life,' the specialist returned from his celestial orbit and smiled at us. Then he handed me a plastic specimen jar. 'Do the tests and then we'll see.'

The mystery of no life in our case, I thought, but we said 'thank you' and Martha took the various forms that she would need to take to the various departments of the hospital over the next few weeks so we could have the various tests that might, just might, show exactly what was stopping us having a baby.

I have to say men get it easy. We just have to masturbate. Martha had to do a hospital decathlon, waiting around at numerous clinics so someone could stick something on, in or up her – all of which had to be done without telling work. I mean, what do you say to your trendy media bosses?

'So we're having some fertility problem.'

'Oh, er, right.'

'I'll probably need some time off.'

'Any idea how much?'

'No, not really. It's kind of open-ended. Could go on for years.'

'Right. Great.'

'Until we have a kid, I guess.'

'And you'll want some more time for that, I suppose…'

My sample should have been light relief in the whole process, but it turned out sex was not the only thing I had problem scheduling. Cursing myself for not inserting 'sperm production' into the BlackBerry, I considered my options on the 11.45 from Cardiff Central. It was turning into a wank against time.

Enforced masturbation against the clock in a public space was not a challenge I had faced before. I do not recommend it. I have masturbated in some quite extraordinary places in my youth, against great odds, occasionally with an almost supernatural poise, so a quick 'job' on a train should have presented no problem. But this time I panicked. I couldn't get an erection in the toilet – the bowl was full of what looked like an unravelled Egyptian mummy who had had an 'accident'. I tried sneaking into first class but ran straight into the ticket inspector. He gave me a dirty look.

'Have you got a ticket?'

'Actually I just need to go to the toilet.'

'These are the first-class toilets.'

There was no use discussing my needs with the man. He looked so miserable I suspected he had never masturbated in his life.

In the end I did it. The perverted will ask how. The truly perverted will probably guess, but I leave it to your imagination. I will only say it was one of the most dexterous pieces of self-stimulation you will ever not witness. If wanking ever came out from under the bed sheets and became an Olympic sport, I would be the Usain Bolt of the discipline.

I gingerly wrapped the specimen jar in a little plastic sandwich bag, then wrapped that in an M&S bag and then stuffed it inside my man bag. I don't know why; this is not the way to store sperm. The correct place for semen in a jar is apparently directly onto your skin, clasped to your bosom, not suffocating inside an airtight plastic bag for several hours. These are the kinds of basic things they should tell you when handing over the jar.

Perhaps I was worried about crime; all those signs at train stations, warning of pickpockets. They annoyed me, those signs. Police arresting wrongdoers, that's what's required. Not signage. Why do people in authority have an unwavering belief in the power of stating the obvious? A town is flooded and the first thing put up is a sign with the words: WARNING: DANGER OF FLOODS!

'Sorted,' the folk-in-charge say.

'How so? It's just a sign saying what happened.'

'Exactly. All sorted...'

Luckily, the retail value of my sperm was probably limited – I can't imagine it would be a popular item to fence down the pub.

'So I've got a *Star Wars: Attack of the Clones* DVD and some bloke's jizz. A fiver for each.'

'Man, I've only got five quid – how do I choose?'

Still, you cannot be too careful with your own sperm and this current batch had been hard earned. I wasn't taking any chances as I tightened the buckles, securing my sample against the dangers of London.

The train finally arrived at Paddington. I walked out into a cool September afternoon, went through the gates, and hopped into a taxi. An hour later, and £40 poorer, I was in front of the The Wicked Witch. She was eating chocolates.

'I've got my sample,' I said, watching as she masticated on a nougat surprise.

'Too late.' A sly, contented smile came across her face as she pointed to a clock on the wall. She smelled victory – another couple's chance of reproducing foiled! But something about the act of semi-public masturbation – the only activity my reproductive organs had been allowed in the past forty-eight hours – had changed me. The remnants of my masculinity were stashed in my bag and whatever happened, someone was going to have a closer look at them.

'I have sperm,' I began, fiddling with the clasp on my bag. 'I produced this sperm under some very harsh conditions. Now either a trained professional can examine it,' I paused. 'Or you can.'

Her smile waned a fraction. I wondered whether I had taken things too far. Was sperm an offensive weapon? Was it legal to threaten someone with your own reproductive juices? Whatever the answer, I'm sure The Wicked Witch understood what a desperate man was willing to do with his own semen.

'Other room,' she conceded, turning her back on me.

For some reason, South Morden's fertility clinic had two waiting rooms; an initial sorting pen and then a smaller room with about six chairs. This, I assumed, was what she meant by the 'other room'. The point of this twofold waiting system was unclear; perhaps it was symbolic of the sperm's journey through the vagina (outer waiting room) into the uterus (inner sanctum) before finally making it to the consultant's room (ovaries).

I could have been reading too much into it.

I certainly had plenty of time to do so. An hour passed. I waited for someone to call my name, or even Martha's, which I was used to being called by now. My sperm and I spent an hour next to a nervous couple, clearly awaiting some important announcement regarding their fertility future. Every few minutes the man would pat his partner's knee and say: 'not long now, not long.'

After the fourteenth 'not long now', I went back to The Wicked Witch. She had finished grazing her way through the chocolates and was now helping herself to a generous slice of lemon sponge.

'Look, I've been waiting a while.'

'Just wait in the other room.'

'Am I on a list or something?'

'No list, just wait in the room!'

I went back. The couple had disappeared. I waited another thirty minutes but no one came. Finally, I stood up. Now I really was ready to kill someone with my sample, however long that might take, but there was no one around. So, in desperation, I did what I have never done before – I broke the rules. I went into the consultants' area without being called. I just did it; I stepped over an invisible line and shuffled into the corridor, willing someone to stop me and my sperm from finding whoever I and my sperm needed to find.

Two footsteps in, there was a door. On the door was a piece of paper with 'Embryology' printed on it. In Comic Sans. I paused. Embryology sounded about right. Those bastard embryologists, I thought, leaving me and my sperm hanging around for hours while they're off flirting with each other down the local Wetherspoon's, laughing at the 'inferts'.

Furious, I threw the door open, or least pushed firmly against it. Inside was a small laboratory and sitting on a stool, staring at me, was a youngish man in a white coat. The embryologist, I presumed. He didn't look like he'd been down the pub. He didn't look very happy at all. To be specific, he didn't look happy with me.

'Mr Cossey?' he asked.

'Yes.'

He looked at the clock on the wall.

'You're late.'

This seemed unfair.

'I've been here for hours. The Wi… the receptionist told me to wait in the other room.'

'This is the other room,' he said shaking his head. His tone suggested it wasn't the first time this had happened. 'This is what she meant by the other room.'

There was a silence. Then he asked:

'Have you got your sample?'

I removed the M&S bag from my man bag, untied it, pulled out the sandwich bag, opened it, pulled out the jar and placed it on the bench. The embryologist picked it up, examined the name, and pushed a clipboard over to me.

'You need to sign,' he said.

I did so, then stood around packing my various bags away, trying to see if there were other samples I could compare mine to. There was nothing. Finally, the embryologist waved a hand towards the door.

'You can go now.'

I went back to the reception and demanded to see The Wicked Witch, but she was on her break from keeping the confectionary industry in business. I vented my fury at one of her sidekicks.

'She told me to go to the other room.'

'That's right. The other room.'

'But how was I supposed to know there was another other room?'

'You went to the other other room?'

'No, I went to the other room, but I needed to go to the other other room.'

'Well, there's your problem right there...'

The conversation was going nowhere. I stormed out of the Portakabin and waited for the bus home. Buses from the South Morden were not a common occurrence, and as I stood there I began to grow nervous. For the first time my sexual prowess, my fecundity, was going to be literally under the microscope. That nerdy embryologist was probably at this very moment staring at my semen, determining whether I was a stud or a dud.

Soon I would know for certain whether I could be a father or not.

I went home and poured myself a manly glass of rosé, ordered a pizza and sat down to watch *University Challenge*. What if I was shooting blanks? Would my wife still love me knowing I had no chance of reproducing?

I tried to put myself in her shoes, but stopped after I'd dumped myself, bought an eighties aerobics leotard and a Walkman and gone off with a six-foot-three corporate lawyer named Kev.

It was all because Martha wasn't home. I didn't like it when Martha wasn't home, but she had disappeared that night to some media party in the West End. I imagined all those fertile young media types strutting around in their trendy shoes, looking like they could reproduce any second.

'God,' I cried. 'Please give me sperm. Please give me millions of sperm. Please don't let me be a dud.'

But God, as usual, was silent on the matter.

Martha got home later and slipped into bed.

'How'd it go?' she asked.

'Oh fine,' I said, but I wasn't so sure. Maybe things weren't going to be fine at all.

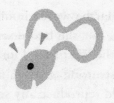

Chapter 7

Results All Round

The results weren't a complete disaster. There were, for example, lots of sperm. Sadly, due to the delay in getting them under the microscope, most of them were dead. This is known as necrozoospermia, which just goes to show that the medical profession doesn't take reproduction seriously. They just made up some terminology in the eighties after smoking spliffs in an Amsterdam movie house.

'Isn't *Necrozoospermia* a film?'

'Nope. It's our new name for dud nuts. You're thinking of *C.H.U.D. – Cannibalistic Humanoid Underground Dwellers.*'

'No, I'm sure we got stoned and then saw something about bloodsucking inseminators called the Necrosperm and who live in an intergalactic zoo...'

The rest of my 'output', according to the embryologist's report, was just lazy.

'Lazy?' I asked, now feeling quite insulted by the whole thing.

'Some of the laziest we've ever seen.' The consultant looked down at the ground as if I had committed some grave crime against manhood.

'Is lazy sperm an actual medical term?'

'Yep.'

I felt they were giving my sperm a moral dimension I wasn't sure they possessed. Were my sperm fraudulently claiming incapacity benefit? Did they keep holding out for a 'real job', complaining that it wasn't worth their while slaving at the coalface of conception? I imagined my sperm down the job centre.

'Look, there's a position here fertilising an egg.'

'It's not really me.'

'You're a sperm. You've got to be realistic.'

'I want something in finance.'

'You live in a scrotal sack. A job in finance isn't for the likes of you. Why don't we give fertilisation a go?'

I begged the doctor to let me produce another sample. To show him what my sperm could do given the right conditions.

'How did you store it?' He asked.

'What?'

'When you were delivering the sample, how did you store it?'

I explained about Cardiff and the M&S bag and the other room. The doctor lifted his hand.

'That would've wiped them out,' he said. 'That's like Spermageddon. You need to keep the jar near your body – in contact with your skin. Didn't anyone tell you?'

A week later a second test proved beyond a shadow of a doubt that I did not have lazy, dead sperm. Well, there were still a few lazy ones, but the rest just tended not to thrive inside a small jar for several hours during a heatwave. I just had sperm that didn't like hanging around.

'Maybe I have impatient sperm,' I suggested.

The doctor laughed.

'Impatient sperm. The very idea! You can have dead sperm, lazy sperm, abnormally shaped sperm or no sperm at all, but you can't have impatient sperm.'

Abnormally shaped sperm? I imagined my freaky, zombie-shaped sperm clambering through the uterus towards Martha's eggs, trying to create a zombie race to take over the world. I imagined Martha and I trying to raise a brood of little zombie babies.

'Brains, brains...' they would cry.

'Ah,' I would say, my arm around Martha, as we looked proudly down at our offspring. 'Their first words...'

'That's not how it works.' The doctor gave me an odd look. 'Abnormally shaped sperm are unable to reproduce. They are a clear sign of male infertility.'

Really? I wondered. What wasn't he telling me? Was my sperm somehow lying inside my testicles, abnormal and impatient, waiting to breed?

'No,' insisted the doctor. 'They're not. They are just lying around not doing very much. You have lazy sperm.'

I was unconvinced. In the future they will discover the impatient sperm gene; the kind of sperm that always wants to get on the plane first, leave the restaurant early and never bothers to finish a job properly.

In other words they could be the executive body running any local council:

'Right, I think that's resolved the pregnancy issue.'

'But we haven't actually inseminated the egg yet.'

'It's five o'clock. I've got to go to a canapés and drinks reception for our "putting poverty first" campaign...'

'The egg is just over there...'

'Sod it.'

Things ticked along. Martha sneaked off from work another half a dozen times to finish her tests, brushing off inquiries into her ongoing medical problem.

And then it was the night before. We lay in bed like young lovers. Well, I was young*ish* and that paunch is posture-related, but anyway use your imagination. We were Lancelot and Guinevere, trying to fall into the sleep of the dead, waiting for the Excalibur of fecundity to be thrust between us.

'The Excalibur of fecundity?' Martha raised an eyebrow. 'What does that mean?'

'Shut up,' I said. Then:

'If it's me,' Martha said, 'you can go.'

'If it's me,' I replied, 'you can't.'

'You're a romantic, Cossey,' she yawned, but we didn't sleep. What would it do to us if one could breed and the other could not? The only conversation we'd had about it was during our first trip to the Morden.

Of course, these talks should've taken place in a supportive and caring environment, with clear signposts and boundaries so we didn't hurt each other. Instead, we began our careful exploration at the back of the bus next to an old drunk with a cough.

'You're not a man, are you?' I asked.

'What?' Martha looked at me suspiciously. The old drunk looked at her suspiciously.

'You know, you're not a guy who's had a sex change and is just too afraid to let me know?'

'You think I'm a man?'

'Well, it would explain the problems we're having.'

Martha thought about it.

'If I was a man, would that make a difference?'

The old man coughed and then nodded, as if to say 'good point, well made'. I was less sure. This was a problem with Martha – you asked her a simple question and she always had to complicate things. She was always turning a straightforward discussion into some kind of existential conundrum, in this instance regarding whether or not I would love my wife if she had once been a man.

'Can't you just say "No, I'm not a man and I have never been one?"'

'But I'm interested,' Martha said, 'as to whether you would still love me if I was a man.'

'Ummm.'

'So you wouldn't love me if I was a man?' Martha turned away in mock horror.

'Of course I'd love you,' I retorted. 'But I'd love you as a man.'

Martha pondered on these words. The old drunk raised his eyebrows and shook his head.

'So you're gay?' she said.

'No,' I replied. 'That's not what I...'

'Maybe that's why we're not having a baby. Because you're a homosexual. Are you faking orgasms?'

Two months after that conversation, the day of reckoning arrived. Martha and I once again headed off on the long journey to South Morden. We got off the bus and entered the little prefab convent for the results. The Wicked Witch was not there, which was a shame, because at least she was someone to kill if we were told we couldn't have children. A different doctor sat us down. She pulled out our file.

We held our breath. What was it to be? Poor egg production? Low sperm count? Badly taught sex education?

We were an instant away from knowing whether one or both of us could not have a child. The hologram of Mrs Skeletor appeared before me again.

Do you really want this? Do you?

'Your results,' the consultant began. Then she waited for the drum roll, *The X Factor*-final pause, and then added that long moment between 'aim' and 'fire' for effect.

'Can you not do that?' I said finally.

'Oh, sorry,' she said. 'Your results are normal.'

Normal. Except for some sperm suffering from mild ennui, everything was normal. Martha's tubes were healthy, ovulation excellent, no diseases of any sort, no HIV, type 2 syphilis or hepatitis. Even her blood pressure was perfect. There was nothing wrong, no reason why we couldn't have a baby. The doctor looked up and smiled.

'It's like this in about fifty per cent of cases,' she said, going on to explain exactly how baffling it all is, this pregnancy malarkey.

We sat there, silent. Something horrible, once again, had been forestalled, delayed. We were back at square one, the essence of our future still unknown. We looked at each other for a moment, just to check. Just to agree on what was next.

'When can we start treatment?' Martha asked.

The doctor shrugged and looked down at her notes. 'There's a waiting list…' It was a long waiting list, and it was unlikely we'd be seen anytime soon.

I began to get the sense that the NHS thought having a baby was really a lifestyle thing and not a medical matter. Why should they help? After all, they don't provide medical support for other lifestyle choices, do they?

Well, except smokers. Smokers puff away for forty years (and don't get me wrong, smoking is great – if I wasn't scared of the old lung/heart/amputated limb thing I'd puff like a chimney – you really can't underplay how pleasant a thing tobacco is) and no one shuts the medicine cabinet when they get a little cough. And the same applies to those whose hobbies include drinking, eating fatty foods, and mountain climbing.

No, if you're an overweight, drunk free-climber up K2 and you lose your grip while lighting up, the NHS will treat you like there's no tomorrow, but if you a want a baby, it really, really doesn't want to know. Somehow loving couples wanting to share their good fortune by raising their own child is less worthy than, well, anything.

Somewhere in the NHS there is a list of priorities for care, which goes like this:

1. Children with cancer.
2. Heroes who saved children with cancer from a fire.
(List carries on: 3, 4, 5… until…)

999.   Serial killers with unsightly tattoo on left foot causing them to lose confidence in their own appearance.

1000.   People who can't have babies.

Ten minutes after our consultation finished, we were standing outside, next to a skip, staring at the Portakabin. Leaning against it was a heavily pregnant woman smoking a cigarette. It seemed like a sign. Martha turned to me.

'Can we go to the hospital next to our house instead?' she said.

'Let's do that,' I nodded. At least it would save us the commute and St William's had a good reputation.

So we did. It took some nagging, two rude words, and a letter of complaint, but a month later we convinced our GP that South Morden wasn't for us, and finally got an appointment at St William's.

Martha was in tears. The Wicked Witch had, for the third time, failed to send our paperwork to St William's. If it didn't arrive by the next day, we would miss our slot with the consultant and then it would be another three months' wait for the next. That would mean almost a year had passed from the first visit to the GP, and we were still no nearer to being treated.

'I'll never get pregnant,' Martha wailed. A wailing Martha is a terrible thing. I sat beside her, feeling powerless.

'We will, Boo,' I said. 'We're nearly there.'

'We are not. We're going to have to buy a dog.'

No one was buying no dog. The only people who could possibly want a dog were the children we weren't having or people with hygiene problems. Once I stood next to a man in a yellow jumper at a party:

'Any kids?' I asked.

'Nah,' replied the man. 'But we've got a couple of dogs though. It's like we're practising.'

Practising? For what? If anything wasn't designed to replace the wrenching hole of childlessness, it's a dog. People who say their dog is like a person are just strange. If you catch your teenage child masturbating, for example, you wash the sheets and never talk of it again; you catch the dog, you chop its testicles off. Your child gets ill, you donate your liver to save it; your dog, you take it down the vet.

'Rufus might pull through…'

'No biggie, we're going to get a hamster anyway.'

'We're not buying a dog,' I said, trying to talk her down from doing something rash.

'We are.' Martha's face rested on her fists. 'A big ugly skinny dog with an ugly floppy face and we're going to have to feed it wet food and I won't be able to do that!'

This was true. Martha can't be near jam for example. She recoils at the sight of tomato ketchup. If you were ever in need of seeing my wife retch, you'd simply need to utter the word 'gelatinous'.

The whole thing was now making me angry. Not in a good way, but in a bad-action-film way. Think *The Crucible* meets *Snakes on a Plane*. I was a hybrid Samuel L. Jackson/ Judge John Hathorne, and I was ready to burn some witches. Armed only with my wits, my sangfroid, and two forms of identification (one with my address), I returned to the South Morden for the final time. If I couldn't give life I was sure as hell going to take it. They were going to rue the day they messed with Mark Cossey and his wife's notes.

I stormed into the Portakabin. There was a queue. Etiquette demanded I wait patiently before committing wholesale slaughter on the administration. As I aggressively inched forward, I imagined myself surrounded by large bookcases of medical notes, a wise old knight, and some Nazis. The theme tune to *Raiders of the Lost Ark* was playing in the background. The chief Nazi, played by The Wicked Witch, grabs a set of notes and looks at them. She screams, her face melting before me. The other Nazis flee in terror past Lara Croft, still trying to reach Pandora's box over a puddle of shallow water.

'Are you sure this a big enough pay-off?'

'Just keep stretching, Ange...'

Meanwhile, the knight shakes his head solemnly.

'She chose poorly.'

I look around. In the corner is a humble set of notes... our notes...

I edged ever closer to The Wicked Witch. She could now sense my imminent arrival and the air crackled with tension as we finally came face to face, Caesar vs Pompey, Churchill vs Hitler, Cowell vs Walsh. We stared at each other.

'The notes,' I said.

Time stopped. The coven fell away from their leader. I noticed a shiny new photocopier and fax machine glistening in one corner. The Wicked Witch stood perfectly still, her nonchalant refusal to look up from her appointment book masking her fear...

'Name?' she said, a Jammie Dodger gripped in her hand like a ninja star.

'The notes,' I repeated, slowly.

'Whose notes?'

'You know whose notes. Martha's notes.'

There was a pause, a beat, a brief moment in the universe, and then:

'You're not Martha.'

Words flashed before me: something that rhymed with 'witch' and then something that rhymed with 'clucking bunt clucker'. I appealed to her: I tried emotional blackmail, Aristotelian logic, I threatened to take her to the European Court of Human Rights, but nothing worked. Suddenly I was clad in the uniform of a Roman officer, the seventh legion behind me, and on my command they would unleash...

'No notes,' The Wicked Witch snapped, destroying the seventh and rendering me naked in front of her. I was defeated, her malevolent shadow looming over me, Martha's notes lost forever in time and space. There was only one thing left to do:

I fell to my knees and begged.

'Please,' I clasped my hands together, tears in my eyes. 'Just give them to me.'

Then somehow, someone in the clinic, someone with the ear of the great god Hubris, finally took Martha's notes, lifted a finger and pressed 'send' on the fax machine. Hearing the sudden squeal of a document being sent electronically, The Wicked Witch, so close to her final victory of denying another couple any chance of happiness, screamed and faded from view.

I stood up and rang Martha on the mobile.

'Ding dong, The Wicked Witch is dead,' I said. These were our code words for success.

'Would you stop being horrible to that poor woman. Did you get the notes?'

'I repeat, The Wicked Witch is dead.'

'They haven't called the police, have they?'

A spectral hand appeared next to me, holding something out. It was one of those cheap, cream-coloured plastic cups, and in it was milky tea. Not nice tea, not pleasant-smelling, but tea nonetheless. I looked up. The hand belonged to The Wicked Witch. I couldn't say she smiled, but something in her face cracked as she pushed the cup into my hand.

'Good luck,' she whispered and then quickly turned away. For a moment I regarded it, then put the rim to my lips, and tasted the brown liquid. And you know, it tasted OK. Not bad at all.

For a moment I just sat there, drinking the tea and listening to The Wicked Witch berating some other poor bloke about his sperm sample. Had we actually gotten any further? Nothing was wrong with us, nothing that medical science could see. No one knew why we weren't pregnant. Martha and I were as in the dark as ever.

It was now over two years since we first started trying. If things had been normal our flat would have been full of dirty nappies and red eyes and a hundred other things we didn't know about yet. Most importantly it would have been full of a baby. Instead, our chance of a family, our big chance of happiness, was now dependent on a still-far-from-perfect science. Suddenly, in that waiting room full of people desperately wanting an answer, I didn't. Once again, I didn't want to know whether Martha and I could have a baby. Why couldn't we just carry on forever, just the two of us, happy and in love?

I stared at the people's faces, expecting their collective expression to answer my fundamental question, give away some overwhelming truth about the human condition.

No one looked back. Their heads were bowed towards the floor as if in prayer. As if they had committed some dark sin. As if shame had left them with no one to ask for forgiveness. For a long time no name was called out, no one moved, no one talked. It was – what was it? I struggled for the word, but it took a while to come. Then I knew it.

It was fear.

I thought we had stood up to fear, tested its mettle, and stared it down. But fear had been having a snooze. A nap. Now, waking up, it yawned, sniffed the air and rubbed its eyes. It stood and towered above me, stretching.

Then fear looked down at me and laughed.

I turned away and left. Outside, I threw the cup in the skip and then fled the South Morden for the last time.

PART 2

TRY HARDER

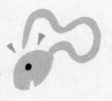

Chapter 8

Artificial Intelligence

The woman rocked back and forth on the plastic chair; her hands were pressed tightly against her ears.

'Turn it off,' she begged. 'Please, for pity's sake, can't they just turn it off...'

Her partner sat in the next seat, clinging to her waist, shouting at another woman standing over them. She, in turn, pointed a remote control at the wall-mounted TV and was pressing the off button repeatedly, but the screen would not die. On it, Jeremy Kyle was berating a pubescent youth dressed in loose tracksuit bottoms and sporting an underdeveloped beard. The strapline underneath read: 'Paul got his girlfriend and her mum pregnant.'

We had arrived at St William's Centre for Reproductive Medicine. We sailed past the sobs and Jeremy's critique of the lad's profligate loins. We landed at reception and checked ourselves in. The noise, the busy waiting room, the fact the clinic was housed in what appeared to be yet another well-hidden Portakabin – none of this touched us.

We'd made it.

'Don't get too excited,' Martha whispered, sitting down, eyes aglow and the word 'excitement' stencilled on her forehead.

'I'm not,' I said. 'I'm not excited.'

I was. I was sick of waiting. I was tired of hiding in the trenches, skulking far from the fertility front line. Finally we were going to see action. We were about to attack the problem head-on with the strongest force known to man. The nuclear bomb of reproductive medicine: *in vitro* fertilisation.

Whatever it was, I knew IVF was the business. For a generation people had spoken these three letters in hushed tones to each other. How so and so's offspring had been teleported into existence by its magic. Now here we were, desperate for some of it. Unleash its power, and in a few months Martha would be pregnant. In less than a year I would be assembling the cot and collapsing the buggy into the boot of the car.

'Martha Cossey?' A consultant appeared, motioning for us to follow him. His accent was Italian. This, I thought, was a good sign; those Italians would know a thing or two about fertility. Turns out no – Italy has a terrible birth rate; their economy is more productive than their bedrooms. That's why they kept voting for Berlusconi, in the forlorn hope he'd improve the population demographic. He certainly had a good crack at it for a pensioner.

The consultant guided us into his office. It was another tiny space, big enough for two but a squeeze for three. What were those architects thinking?

'So what do we need in this room?'

'Well, there's the doctor, and the woman.'

'What about the bloke?'

'Who?'

'You know, the loser who can't get his wife pregnant.'

We squashed in. The Italian pulled out our notes, and began to flick through them.

'Your infertility is unexplained?' he asked. We nodded.

'Your first test was very bad,' he said, waving a finger at me. It was like having a criminal record. You make one mistake, under trying conditions, and it's held against you for the rest of your life.

'What about Cossey for that new senior executive position?'

'What, Two-condom Cossey?'

'The very same.'

Rustling of paper.

'Have you seen this?'

'Dear God, if his sperm's that lazy...'

It wasn't fair. I'd had another test proving the fair to middling virility of my sperm, but no one ever looked at the other test. I willed the consultant to look at the other test, but he flipped through the remaining pages quickly, my unique, impatient but probably earnest sperm once again ignored. Then he closed the notes, satisfied.

'All right,' he said. 'I think we will start on unassisted IUI and see how we do.'

IUI? I looked at Martha. What was unassisted IUI? Was it Latin for IVF? Wasn't IVF already in Latin? I looked back at the doctor.

'Sometimes it is called AI,' he smiled. 'Perhaps you're more familiar with this?'

Like the movie *A.I. Artificial Intelligence*? That sounded positive; the treatment that is, not the film. No one knows what that film was about. The parents get a robot kid to replace their dead kid who isn't really dead and then they dump the robot kid when the dead kid wakes up and then something about a balloon and then aliens.

'The film's not important,' Martha sighed, dragging me back to the subject at hand. She somehow already knew what IUI meant, but asked the consultant to explain it to her husband.

'Of course,' he shuffled his chair around. Our knees touched. 'IUI is short for intrauterine insemination. It's completely straightforward. We wait for your partner to ovulate. Then we take a sample of your sperm and we use a tube and insert it into the upper part of her vagina. Simple.'

Silence. My eyes widened. His gaze relaxed. Martha bit her nails.

'So,' I said, waiting for him to add something more, but his explanation appeared complete.

'So you get my sperm,' I continued.

'Exactly.'

'And then you insert it into Martha.'

'Mmm-hmm.'

'With a tube.'

'*Esatto*!'

Martha noticed something on the floor. She began an earnest study of it.

'Just so you're clear,' my voice went up a semitone. 'That's what we've been doing. For the past two and a bit years I've been inserting sperm into my wife, using my own specially designed, organically grown tube. You may have heard of it, it's called a penis. The reason we're here is because the whole sperm-inserting thing isn't doing the trick.'

The consultant nodded, as if expecting my outburst.

'Ah – but this time an embryologist will do it.'

'What? Have sex with my wife?'

'Ha – if you like, yes.'

I did not like. Where was the bloody IVF? The life-giving holy grail of IVF?

The consultant laughed.

'You don't just jump straight into IVF,' he said. 'This would be like giving a teenager a Ferrari. Let's try the IUI first, OK?'

I slumped back in my chair. He was, after all, the doctor. If he thought inserting my sperm with a little more finesse might do the trick, who was I to argue? If he wasn't worrying about our childless state, why should we? Maybe things weren't as bad as we thought.

Maybe we didn't need IVF.

We returned to reception and joined the queue to get inseminated. There we discovered it would be four weeks before we started on the Ford Escort of fertility treatments, and then another two until some sleazy embryologist had weird hospital sex with Martha.

It was a long wait. Outwardly, I carried on with my usual unflinching stoicism, but the tube sex played on my mind. I became obsessed with how long and wide it might be. How deep would it go? I wanted to discuss my fears with Martha, but this was exactly the sort of thing she would mock me about.

I also realised that, despite past disagreements between my penis and me, and the trying times it had put me through, I wasn't happy about it being superseded. Every time I visualised this competing android phallus, it grew bigger. By the time I confessed my concerns, the Russians were using it to pipe gas through the Ukraine.

'What giant robot penis?' Martha asked, searching for something to cook in the fridge. 'Where do these ideas come from?'

The film *A.I. Artificial Intelligence*, obviously.

'It'll just be a piece of tubing,' she said, making a face at an old limp carrot in the vegetable box.

'Metaphorically,' I said, 'it will be a penis. A penis replacement. *My* penis replacement.'

'It's still your sperm.'

'I'm being castrated.'

Martha shrugged.

'You just need to man up about it.'

I looked at her and the carrot. 'What kind of a man mans up about being castrated?'

'The kind that can't get his wife pregnant,' Martha smiled, throwing the limp vegetable in the bin. 'Now what about sausages for dinner?'

Aside from my upcoming virtual penectomy, things were going well. As ovulation day approached, Martha went to the clinic several times to be scanned, and each time she returned her eyes were a little brighter, she stood a little taller.

'How was it?' I'd ask.

'Good,' she would say. 'Looking good.'

I didn't care what they were scanning for: Xenomorphs, chocolate buttons, the Higgs boson. It didn't matter. What mattered were Martha's eyes and that expectant gleam coming from them. Suddenly all around us was a vibe; a sense that this was going to work: the Cosseys were going to get their baby.

D-Day arrived. The morning was divided into two parts. First, I would produce my sample – St William's luxury Portakabin was a step up from the Morden, and they had a room set aside for this activity, a sort of Virginia Woolf's *A Room of One's Own* but with ejaculations.

After I had made my contribution, my sample would be cleaned and then the second part would commence. My sperm would, through the evil power of the robot penis, somehow be injected into Martha.

Then, nine months later, a baby would appear.

'Nervous?' Martha asked as my name was called out.

'No,' I laughed. Then I met the anti-wank chair.

'I do it on that?' I asked the embryologist.

'Do it where you like,' he shrugged. 'Just lock the door.'

I fidgeted on the chair. Then work rang. This was frustrating, as I hadn't actually taken the day off. It wasn't clear what kind of leave my upcoming activity qualified as. Was I sick? On holiday?

'Mark, your form has "off for a wank" written on it.'

'Yep.'

'You need a whole day?'

I fidgeted some more. Then I noticed the room wasn't soundproof.

It was the footsteps that alerted me. As I sat there, in that demonic chair for the first time, alone with the bad porn collection, I heard slow and deliberate footsteps come down the corridor towards me. Clack, clack, clack they went, moving ever nearer. Were they coming for me, I wondered. Was I in an eighties horror film? Was it Death, arriving to collect my masculinity? If it was, did he know he was too late?

The footsteps paused outside. I clutched my manhood in terror, shielding it from whatever evil was about to befall me. For an aeon nothing happened – someone, something just stood there, waiting. Finally, a shadow passed across the bottom of the door and the footsteps receded: clack, clack, clack.

The air fell from my lungs. I tried to refocus, but my now heightened senses became aware of other noises. Two nurses discussing a patient. The sound of a text message arriving. It was like masturbating in a tent. Not that I'd know. I hate camping; I'm always amazed when people announce their upcoming outdoor adventure.

'Two weeks in France, it's going to be great to get away from it all.'

Away from what? Sanitation? Every single person who goes camping just ends up in a motorway hotel eating stale sandwiches talking about how next year's holiday must include a roof and a toilet. I despised tents, and I despised masturbating in one.

Still, I needed to get on. Once again I wiggled in the chair.

Then I considered the fact that sound, after all, was a two-way thing. If I could hear them, then they could hear me. I pondered the aural qualities of self-gratification. Was I completely silent during the process? I didn't moan, did I?

Someone would definitely hear a moan. What about a grunt? Would these flimsy walls muffle a grunt?

Some subdued and self-conscious moments later, I emerged, slightly shaken, specimen in hand. I found the door marked 'Embryology'. I knocked gingerly.

'Come in,' said a female voice.

'Really?' I said.

'Really,' the voice snapped.

I opened the door. An attractive young woman stood in front of me. I held out my sperm roughly at the height of her breasts, wondering what to say.

'Howdy,' I said. *Howdy?*

'You can put your sample there.' Her emotionless face nodded at the bench. Of course I could. Leave the fruit of my loins, a less than abundant crop, in a room with a twenty-something blonde. Where's the problem?

'You'll need to sign for it,' she said, snapping surgical gloves over her hands.

I went and sat next to Martha.

'The embryologist was a woman,' I whispered.

'No?' Martha feigned astonishment.

'Why would a woman want to work with men's sperm?'

'I don't know, man-from-the-1950s. Why do male gynaecologists want to look at women's bits all day?'

Good point. Why do men chose a career in women's genitalia? Surely it would put you off the whole thing. You poke around down there all day and then you come home and your wife demands some further poking and then it's time to get up and start again.

Still, things were on the up. Martha was ovulating, my sperm was being supercharged, and we were on the cusp of our first attempt at a medically assisted conception. Even Jeremy Kyle was having a day off paternity stories and was shouting at a transsexual for lying to his/her husband instead. All the signs were positive as we followed the nurse out of reception and towards destiny.

She led us straight to a supply cupboard.

'Sorry,' she said. 'We don't have anywhere else to get changed.'

No doubt there is a limit to the kind of talent you can get to work on Portakabin design, but come on: no changing rooms? For the patients?

Amongst the packets of surgical gloves and swabs, Martha got undressed and then we put on our gowns and pulled on our paper shoes. Alone for a moment, we looked at each other.

'Ready?' Martha asked.

We kissed. That was one thing the giant artificial penis wouldn't be able to do to my wife. They couldn't take that away from us.

'Ready?' the nurse interrupted, slightly taking it away.

We entered the dimly lit theatre. I searched for the mechanical sex organ, but it clearly hadn't been wheeled in yet. Then the low sounds of an animal in pain started to fill my ears. For a moment I thought they hadn't removed the last patient and were being euphemistic in describing IUI as mildly uncomfortable.

I looked to the nurse.

'Whale songs,' she smiled, proudly pointing at a speaker built into the wall. 'We find it very relaxing for the patients.'

'Sperm whales?' I smiled.

'Humpbacks, I think,' she yawned.

Touché. As the sea mammals continued to groan atonally in the background, the nurse produced a jar from the fridge. She held it up to Martha.

'Is this your partner's sperm?'

Martha took the jar, unsure what to do. I imagine most sperm looks similar. I don't believe I'd be able to identify my sperm in a sperm line-up, but I studied the jar to see if there were any telltale signs confirming its provenance. Then Martha brought it into the light.

'This sperm,' she said, 'is pink.'

Indeed it was. It was the bright, luminescent pink of Pepto-Bismol. It looked almost radioactive as it glowed in its own luxuriant rosy pinkness.

'My sperm isn't pink,' I said.

'Oh no,' laughed the nurse. 'We do that. We make it pink.'

'Why?' I asked. Why would they do that?

I imagined my luminous pink sperm racing into Martha, desperately trying to keep a low profile to avoid the antibodies placed there to kill them.

'Are we going to be OK?' one sperm would ask nervously.

'Sure,' Sperm Leader would reply, slapping his fellow sperm on the back. 'It's like we've got camouflage.'

'Actually the interior of the vagina is more of a brownish pink,' piped a third sperm.

'And camouflage doesn't normally glow.'

Elsewhere, two antibodies shake their heads sadly.

'Would you look at this,' Antibody Number One would say, as my brave luminous sperm attempted an inconspicuous shuffle towards the uterus.

'Well,' said Antibody Number Two as he cracked his knuckles, 'we've gotta kill them, but it's not cricket.'

'Pink's good,' the nurse beamed, taking the jar back off Martha, who agreed that the name on it was mine, regardless of what was inside.

The embryologist arrived. He was a tall, gangly, chipper chap called Geoffrey. Of course he was chipper, I mused, he was having robot sex with hundreds of women.

He nodded hello to me and then gave Martha a big, cheesy grin.

'You know what we're doing today?' he winked. Well, maybe didn't actually wink, but you could see he had been disciplined about winking in the past.

'Whale sex?' Martha suggested.

'Ah yes, good, isn't it? Turn them up a little, will you, nurse.'

The whales got louder. Geoffrey helped my wife onto the trolley.

'First,' he said, attaching stirrups on either side of Martha. 'I am going to take this sperm,' he nodded at the jar. 'And I'm going to use a thin tube to put the sperm inside you. How's that for you?'

A thin tube. I liked the sound of that.

Martha nodded, placing her legs into the stirrups.

Geoffrey opened the jar, and extracted the fruit of my loins into a long skinny piece of tubing. Inside, I laughed; I had been frightened of this? That little thing? I suddenly felt as virile as a man with fertility issues and pink sperm can.

Geoffrey squatted on a stool between my wife's legs, holding the tube like a conductor's stick. There was a pause as if he was waiting for the orchestra to settle.

'Nurse,' he said. 'Lights please.'

The lights dimmed. It sounded like the whales had encountered some Japanese fishermen doing 'research' and Martha and I were having a foursome with two people we didn't know; but it would all be worth it when we held our beautiful baby. Plus, she wasn't being inseminated by an artificial penis at all. I squeezed her hand.

'Maybe this time we'll get our little Ripley?' I whispered.

Martha squeezed back.

'We're not calling it Ripley,' she said.

The tube went in. There was a pause and then, with the quiet satisfaction of a job well done, Geoffrey withdrew.

'OK,' he smiled. 'Now we wait.'

We were grateful. Something had happened. A procedure, an operation, a thing. We thanked Geoffrey and the nurse; we complimented them on their whales and their colour choices and the smooth insertion. We left the clinic with a spring in our step.

Later that night, Martha slipped into bed shivering from a cold bath. We held each other and I thought: *this is going to work*.

The clinic had told us to wait two weeks before taking the pregnancy test. This is because the NHS bought all their testing kits in the 1960s when it actually took that long to confirm conception. Now the science of testing urine is so advanced you can confirm a pregnancy weeks before actual intercourse, but as I was going to America for work, we agreed to wait the full fourteen days.

'I'll miss you,' Martha said as I lifted my bag.

'Get pregnant,' I ordered.

Martha saluted and then I was in a car going towards Heathrow.

Five days later it was early morning in downtown LA. I was watching the production team of *Heroes* turn a street into New

York, looking on in wonder at the speed in which the location became full of yellow taxis and green street signs. The show was already the hottest thing in the States, and was on its way to becoming an international hit which the BBC had just acquired.

My mobile rang. It was Martha.

'It's negative,' she said.

I didn't need to ask what.

'I thought…'

'I'm not pregnant.'

'OK. Love you.'

'Yeah. Love you too.'

Martha hung up. The Californian sun beamed down. I was about to see the future Mr Spock in action. An instant before I had been excited; I was in the epicentre of the creative world, watching some of the biggest names in showbiz, looking eagerly on as Zachary Quinto walked out of a New York convenience store, his character searching for another victim.

I felt empty. Sick. For ten days I had held out real hope that our problem would be solved, that somehow the medical world would charm us up a baby. Now, for the first time, there it was, clear as the Californian sun: the fact we might never have a child. Never. No matter what.

Then there was something else: a dry dusty taste started to fill my mouth, its odd texture reminding me of something. In my head I heard the muffled cries of a child…

The director's hand went up.

'OK.' He stood up, shaking his head. 'We'll do another take.'

The dryness passed. The world returned and it was time to go home. I picked up my man bag and said goodbye to our producer. I got in a taxi which took me to the wrong hotel. I argued with the driver, but he couldn't understand me. Then I rang Martha and we argued, and she didn't understand me. Then I stormed out into West Hollywood, disappointed with myself, furious at another failed production and my part in it.

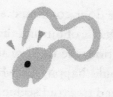

Chapter 9

North London
Restaurant
Incident

Martha was coiled up on our sofa, jeans around her knees, hissing with pain. Dark bruises marked her thighs and spots of fresh blood mixed in with spilled tea from a fallen mug on the Xthorp rug. I stood above her, syringe gripped between my thumb and two fingers, the needle red, surveying the chaos.

Someone was knocking at the door.

'Any better?' I asked.

'Some,' she whimpered, rubbing the latest wound. 'Anyway, I asked for it.'

This was true. Our living room now resembled a scene of domestic violence. Over the past week I had repeatedly assaulted Martha with a sharp object and she had accepted the attacks without protest, agreeing I had no choice and proving the old proverb was true: you do always hurt the ones you love.

The knocking at the door continued.

Some men get a kick out of hurting their spouses. Witnessing the pain and humiliation, the thrill of using violence to wield power. Not me. I would happily tie Martha up, gag her, and put a bag over her head to avoid seeing her upset.

'But that would make me upset,' Martha objected.

'Yes,' I agreed. 'But at least I wouldn't see it.'

Martha grimaced and offered me a hand. I pulled her up off the sofa and held her steady for a moment, then she pulled her jeans up and limped off to the bedroom; her crippled demeanour proof I was no natural in the world of intramuscular injection.

For the third time someone knocked. I opened the door.

'Tesco's,' a man croaked; a trolley of groceries in front of him. He noted the syringe in my hand.

'Did you order Tesco's?' I called out to Martha.

'Yes,' she cried back, her voice still wavering.

I turned back to the man.

'You'd better come in.'

The Tesco man was not happy about coming in. His happiness receded further when he noticed the assorted packets of needles, vials and other injecting accoutrements sitting on our table. He shivered slightly.

'Cold outside?' I asked.

'Sort of,' he nodded, eyes darting around.

'It's OK,' I waved a hand over our drug stockpile. 'We're trying for a baby.'

'Oh,' he smiled, searching for a response. 'We're out of pizzas.'

Tesco's left. I put the used syringe into the yellow hazardous-waste bucket that sat next to the tinned tomatoes. I began to pack away the groceries. I wondered who was to blame for this mess.

Mime was to blame, I decided. It was all mime's fault.

I'd returned from LA six weeks earlier to the news that St William's was proposing another round of IUI. I nodded, hoped for the best and waited for the worst. For the second time Martha and I entered the procedure room, listened to the whales, and watched my pink sperm disappear.

Later that evening, I discovered Martha's abdomen covered in oily goo.

'Dry skin?' I asked.

She shook her head.

'Progesterone cream.'

My finger touched her moist belly.

'It's supposed to help.' Martha sounded dubious.

It helped. It helped explain what Bon Jovi meant by 'Slippery When Wet'. It helped Martha experience her first major outbreak of acne. What it didn't do was get her pregnant. Ten days later she emerged from the toilet.

'Negative?' I asked.

Two sad little nods.

'How do you feel?'

'Slimy.'

We went back to the clinic. They wanted to update us on our progress. I don't know why. They could have just sent us a blank email with the word 'none' in the subject heading. Geoffrey the embryologist, despite his creams and coloured semen, his titrations and his aquatic mammals, had failed us. I was frustrated. Martha was frustrated. Surely it was time for IVF? I promised myself that I wasn't taking no for an answer.

Then we met Nurse Ratched.

How she had arrived at St William's from a 1960s novel set in a mental asylum in Oregon I don't know. She should be dead, or at least very old, but the resemblance was striking; perhaps she was a ghost, a beautiful white wraith, the spirit of Nurse Ratched.

Perhaps she was the undead Nurse Ratched.

'So,' she commenced, the tainted smile of the damned painted across her face. 'How do you feel things are going?'

It must be a spirit-world thing, the asking of pointless questions, but how did we feel? Did it matter? Conception wasn't an opinion. There wasn't an emotional spectrum of embryo existence and no one sent you a card for almost having a baby. Pregnancy either 'was' or 'was not'.

And we was not.

'Well,' Martha said. 'I'm not pregnant.'

Ratched studied the notes.

'But you are ovulating, which is good.'

'I've ovulated since puberty,' Martha rejoined.

'… and there's a reasonable amount of sperm.'

Reasonable? Reasonable wasn't a good word. Reasonable went on your work appraisal after you'd set fire to a colleague. Couldn't she say 'overwhelming'? Or 'more than sufficient'? Did it have to be 'reasonable'?

'Reasonable?' I challenged.

'Reasonable,' she confirmed, smoothing a wisp of hair.

'And yet,' Martha steered the conversation back to its purpose. 'I'm still not pregnant.'

Nurse Ratched sniffed the air. She smelled trouble. Once again, here were the living, crying out for a baby and yet daring to question her.

'We should try one more round of unassisted IUI,' she said, smiling, her eyes meeting Martha's.

Martha smiled back. There was a smile-off.

'The thing is,' Martha said, rubbing her chin. 'I'm not pregnant.'

A slightly sinister, unrelenting tone entered her voice. To my experienced eye, Martha was letting everyone know that she was up for a fight, that the fight would not be pleasant, and wouldn't it be better all round if we just did what she said. She leaned in closer.

'We need to move on,' she said.

Nurse Ratched retreated a little, glancing at me.

'And you, Mark. How do you feel?'

I let my hand drop beside me. It found Martha's. Our fingers gripped.

'IVF 'em,' I said. 'Let's nuke the bastards.'

Martha coughed, reminding me that nuclear talk was special to the two of us; that we weren't to discuss the atomic, chemical, or conventional annihilation of people, things or reproductive organs in public.

'I mean let's move on,' I agreed.

'Fine.' Nurse Ratched turned to her computer. Now I smiled. Had the forces of good won a victory? Had the crucifix of Martha's righteous anger forced the hand of the undead? 'We'll try assisted IUI.' She clicked her mouse twice.

'Assisted?' I asked, but Nurse Ratched pretended not to hear.

'Assisted?' I turned to Martha, but she was already standing up to leave.

Where was my IVF?

We left the clinic and started to walk home.

'Assisted?' I asked again, stopping Martha in a quiet back alley behind the hospital. 'What does that mean? Some kind of pump for the sperm dildo? Aquatic mammal sex beamed directly onto our retinas?'

'Medically assisted,' Martha punched me in the shoulder. 'They're going to use drugs to help me ovulate.'

'I thought you were a good ovulator?'

'This is true. I am a top ovulator.' Martha blushed with pride at her excellent ovulation skills.

Martha's Achilles heel, her kryptonite, was the compliment. She could no more resist a kind word than Prince Harry a kind, naked, girl. She was the human equivalent of a sheet of Plenty kitchen roll, with the ability to absorb far more positive feedback than the average person. Give her praise and her brain turns to progesterone goo.

'But if you're the ultimate ovulating machine,' I continued. 'What good are ovulating drugs going to do?'

Martha stopped.

'I think…' she considered the question, '… it's diagnostic.'

Diagnostic? Surely the diagnosis was straightforward. We had no child. We were childless. Weren't we onto the cure bit now? Maybe St William's suspected that we weren't actually trying and were testing us. It was true that the question of sex had never come up since our first visit to the GP, and during the whole process no one had ever asked: had we done it? Surely it was worth putting on a form as a simple, multiple-choice question? An easy-to-understand 'Have you ever had intercourse? Yes/No/Don't know?' Then the consultant could be sure:

'Well, the tests all seem fine.'

'Brilliant!'

'Look, I know it's silly but...'

'Go on.'

'Well, you've ticked 'no' to sex.'

'That's right.'

'I see. Not interested in intercourse as a means of conception?'

'Tried it once. Nasty business.'

An uncomfortable pause.

'Quite. And yet traditionally we like the couple to have a go first...'

'Roo,' Martha stopped me. 'They don't think we're celibate. They just want us to try the drugs first.'

I ended my protest. After all, I did have a soft spot for drugs. There should be a religion for drugs. You would never be disappointed in the Church of Drugs.

'Oh, lord of drugs, take away my pain...'

'No worries,' a stoned drug-priest would say, pumping morphine into your arm. 'How's that?'

Of course there are side effects. Lung cancer, gun crime, prostitution, that moment when a friend of your parents suddenly asks you if you'd like some really formidable 'skunk', causing you profound inter-generational embarrassment. Still, on the whole, drugs have done the human race proud. What harm could a few fertility pills do?

'They're not pills,' Martha muttered.

No pills then. My mind skipped through the other methods of drug-taking. A spray? A patch? Surely not an enema? Or even a douche? For some reason I imagined we'd end up settling on a douche.

'Injections,' Martha whistled. 'Lots of injections.'

Injections. Martha didn't like injections. Or blood. In fact, pretty much anything to do with human biology was off-limits. She couldn't even write the words 'bile' or 'marmalade' without feeling queasy, all of which was a disability now she was working on the TV medical drama *Holby City*.

'How do you watch it?' I asked.

'With a bucket – and I turn away at the gory bits.'

Martha would never be able to inject herself, but if not her, then who?

'You,' Martha said. 'You, you idiot.'

Two days later we were back at the clinic in front of a new nurse. I hadn't thought of a name for her yet; she wore one of those multicoloured, braided bracelets that were fashionable around the millennium and had messed-up hair that was possibly cool in the eighties; I know this because it still looked good to me. I began to imagine her in a film with Michael Douglas, maybe dressed in a pressed, white shirt and nothing else.

Nurse Injecty? I thought. Nurse Hair, New York Hippy Nurse? Nothing seemed to stick. She remained, at present, just Nurse.

'Right,' she said. 'Have either of you had any experience with intramuscular injections?'

I considered the question. I'd once seen a friend get a tattoo of Kermit the Frog. Did that count? The nurse shook her head.

'We'll start you on Gonal-f.' She began to click her mouse.

I snorted.

'Something funny?' she asked, her face earnest, studied. She could see nothing wrong with the name Gonal-f, but please. Gonal? F? Asthmatics, for example, get Ventolin – just the name makes it easier to breathe. Hay fever sufferers get the Swiss Alps of Clarytin, and even a simple headache tablet gets the powerful, head-soothing Nurofen.

We got Gonal. We got the words 'gonad' and 'anal' rammed together with a grade 'F' attached to it.

'It requires a daily injection into the muscles of either the thigh or the buttock...' the nurse continued.

Then she paused. As if something had just occurred to her. As if she had discovered some inner self, some divine inspiration. She straightened her back, ran her hands through her hair until progress was halted by the knots, then relaxed her shoulders.

'Would you like a demonstration?' She stared intently at us.

We nodded eagerly. I thought we might get a video, or a PowerPoint presentation, or even a practical, in the flesh, show-and-tell.

Instead, we got mime. Nurse Mime.

The sudden presentation of her straightened palms, flat against an imaginary horizontal, should have been a hint, but we were in a hospital, not a fringe festival in southern France. The hand movements that followed provided few clues that we were witnessing an unrehearsed example of the lowest form of performance art. Later, Martha claimed to understand Nurse Mime's interpretation of wiping an invisible buttock with an imaginary swab. There was definitely something about cleaning a blackboard, but what those final flourishes signified will forever be a mystery.

The performance came to an end.

'All clear?' smiled Nurse Mime, lowering the tools of her trade.

We shook our heads slowly.

'Then,' she continued, using actual words, 'before ovulation you'll need to inject the hCG trigger shot, and this gets a bit complicated.'

The palms of her hands once again stood erect before us.

'Let me show you…'

It was like a mute Heston Blumenthal teaching you how to stuff a chicken. My mind began to wander. Was there no other way to learn the art of injecting a human being?

We went home with our drugs and our needles and syringes, and an incredibly vague idea of what to do with them. If the injections did little to help regulate Martha's already regular ovulations, they did provide a painful daily reminder of our own reproductive failure as a couple. Up until this point we had often been able to forget our troubles. For days at a time, we lived in peace, watched a comedy, met friends. Felt normal.

Now, each evening, our own barrenness came back to haunt us in the form of the needle. Every night Martha pulled her trousers down, offered up some flesh, and turned away, waiting for my mime-trained attack.

Then a text arrived. It was from the Morgans; they had finally discovered a babysitter in the form of Sarah's mother and wanted to go out for dinner. A night of freedom, as they called it, without the babies.

We hadn't seen them since the obligatory visit to inspect the twins. I remembered it well. Proud father greeting us at the door. Pram in the hallway. Glowing mother holding cherubs one and two, both sleeping like angels. Cards on the bookshelf and the vague smell of antiseptic cream mixed in with something else.

'I'm for not...' I began.

'We're going,' confirmed Martha.

On the big night we had, for logistical reasons, been unable to return home for the nightly stabbing and were now sitting, pensive, in a Pizza Express. Soon the Morgans would arrive for one of their first, post-baby, nights out. Martha had brought the Gonal and the plan was to inject it before they arrived.

'I'll just nip to the loo and do it,' said Martha, all nonchalant bravado.

Off she went. I waited. Drinks arrived. Time passed. Martha returned, sat down, and took a sip of wine.

'Well?' I asked.

Martha shook her head.

'OK,' I said, taking control. I leaned in, motioning for Martha to come closer.

'I'm going to go to the toilet.' I looked over at the waiter. He was, like all his brethren, ignoring me. It's amazing how waiters do that. How do restaurants make money? How does food get served? They just employ people to walk around quickly, avoiding your gaze no matter what. What was I? A basilisk?

'Boo,' Martha interrupted my train of thought. 'No one knows what a basilisk is.'

'It's a mythical creature whose gaze turns people to stone. Lots of people know what it is.'

'Roo,' Martha took my hand. 'What's the plan?'

Of course. The plan.

'I go to the toilet,' I said. 'In a few minutes you get up, come to the toilet, knock three times on the cubicle door, and then I'll stab you.'

Martha looked at me. It was not a positive look, but in the end she nodded. I stood up.

'Remember,' I whispered. 'Three times.'

'No one knocks on a cubicle door,' Martha waved me off. 'We don't need a code.'

I went to the men's. This was unfortunate as Martha went to the women's. That should have been in the plan. Five minutes later we were reunited in front of the toilets.

'Out of courtesy,' Martha said, 'can we use the ladies? It's cleaner.'

We entered the toilets again and locked ourselves in a cubicle. Martha handed me the needle.

She unclipped her belt. She wriggled her jeans just low enough to expose her buttocks. For a moment I considered the fact that my wife had fine buttocks. Then I wondered if it was a bit pervy, staring at my wife's soon-to-be-stabbed buttocks, in a toilet, in a restaurant. Finally, I attached the needle to the syringe and held up the vial of Gonal.

Then someone knocked on the door. Three times.

We froze. I looked at Martha. *Who else knew the code?* Then there was a voice.

'Please,' it said. 'Please come out.'

We remained silent. At that moment I wished I'd never been born, let alone trying to help the next, clearly reluctant, generation. I looked at the syringe, now half full of medicine, then down at Martha's exposed flesh.

'Please,' the voice said again. 'Come out.'

It was no use. If Martha screamed, the voice would probably call the police, so she pulled up her jeans, tucking away her still unstabbed bottom, and we opened the door. There was the waiter, staring at us. Now, I thought bitterly, now you want to start making eye contact with the customer.

'You cannot be in here,' he said.

'You don't understand…' I began to explain.

'I understand, but you cannot do that here,' he said, pointing us back towards the restaurant.

He escorted us out of the women's toilets and back to our table. Standing next to it, pulling off their jackets, were the Morgans. Their faces worn, bags under their eyes, ashen-skinned.

'Oh, for God's sake,' Martha whispered. 'What do we do now?'

The four of us greeted each other as normal: cheek kisses, hugs, a manly handshake, but we were all hiding something. It was like a Christmas dinner on *EastEnders*, emotions simmering underneath, secrets ready to burst out and destroy all human kinship…

Five minutes later, as we all considered the menu, Martha squealed.

'Are you all right?' Sarah asked.

'Fine, fine,' Martha squeaked. 'Something just went down wrong. That's all.'

The waiter shot me a suspicious glance, but he could go to hell. Underneath the table I had finally managed to stab Martha, in a pizza restaurant, and I had got away with it.

'How are the babies?' I asked, relaxing.

Their response was an instant too slow, the delay allowing their eyes to briefly meet, a conspiratorial glance. Then Steve looked at me, dark circles under his eyes.

'Wonderful,' he said. 'They're both great.'

Our pizzas arrived. For the first time in my life, I regarded an American Hot without enthusiasm. What was happening? I looked around me, everyone was just picking at their food. Something was wrong. Pizza-hating wrong.

Later, as we carried the half-asleep Morgans out to a taxi, Steve turned to me.

'I can't do it,' he said. 'I just can't.'

We stopped. I couldn't answer. What he was going through was the very life change we so desperately wanted. I examined his face in the neon of the restaurant sign: it was deprived of sleep, of blood, of oxygen; there was a nick where he had cut himself shaving.

'Sorry.' Steve rubbed his cheeks, tortured by the unending noise and light around him. 'I know you guys are trying – don't let me put you off. It'll be worth it. A hundred times worth it.'

His voice sounded unconvinced. A minute later we waved them off, got the next cab and began the journey home.

'Sarah OK?' I asked.

'Depressed,' Martha replied. 'Twins sounds tough.'

She rubbed her thigh. Then she asked the question we were both thinking:

'Why are we doing this?'

She pulled down the window, and the chilled night air rushed into the car. The taxi drove down the Archway

Road towards London, its skyline calling us home to our empty flat where I thought – I hoped – some kind of answer awaited us.

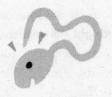

Chapter 10

Do You Really Want It?

'Why' is the worst house guest – just ask any philosopher. Nietzsche asked Why in for coffee and got syphilis off a horse. Socrates asked and then it was hemlock time. David Beckham probably can't spell the word and he's rich and beautiful and everyone loves him.

And the Schwarzenegger of whys? It's this: why have a baby? It's the quizzical equivalent of running over a gypsy in a Stephen King novel; no good will come from it.

Our flat turned into the set of *Newsnight*. Paxman sat before us, spitting out questions: why did we want children? Did we want to be gods? Were we just sheep, following others? Why were we suffering for something that didn't even exist? Why, why, why?

He had a point. The bits of parenthood I'd witnessed were like the plot of a Wes Craven film. No freedom, no sleep, no help, followed by endless screaming and constant exposure to grotesque body fluids.

Then you die.

Did I even like children? I wondered. I'd never spent more than an hour or two with them at a time. The offspring of our friends didn't fill me with strange, potent emotions. I would make an awful nursery assistant.

Why on earth did we want a baby?

I left home to its epistemological nightmares and went to work. It was there I had my first real conversation with Mrs Skeletor. We had a meeting about a project we were working on and found ourselves booked into an airless cupboard down in the basement of Television Centre; following the BBC rule that the more important an appointment was, the more prison-like the accommodation had to be.

So there we sat, feeling moderately important and very claustrophobic.

'I need a cigarette,' Mrs Skeletor finally confessed.

We escaped, got coffee and sat outside. She pushed a pack of Marlboro Lights towards me.

'Given it up,' I said.

'Taken it up,' she laughed. I smiled; despite the smoking, she looked tanned, relaxed and healthier than before. She had put on some weight.

'You're not what I expected,' she said.

'No?'

'You're thinner,' she laughed again. Then I noticed a white band of skin around her ring finger.

Do you really want it, do you?

Our meeting ended and I headed towards the tube. Standing in the crowded carriage, I studied my own wedding band. I wondered what kind of marriage the Skeletors had once had.

Were there always cracks in it? Something not quite right? Or had infertility done them in all by itself? Had Why killed their relationship?

I walked home quickly. I opened the door and called out to Martha. No answer. For a moment I panicked – had she left me? Had my brutal injections caused her to see some fatal flaw in our lives together? I called out again and then I noticed it; two bare feet peering out from the kitchen, the heels facing the ceiling.

'Marthalanche,' I cried, rushing forward.

My wife has many skills. The least useful of these is the innate ability to precariously stack heavy cookware in high places. Instinctively, she can pile up layer upon layer of pots and pans into the top cupboard until it evolves into a culinary cliff face, set off by the slightest movement. Having achieved this, she then decides it's time to cook. Then the Marthalanche occurs.

For a brief second, as I took the two or three steps across the hall to the kitchen, I imagined Martha dead. Horrible visions flashed before me: her brain crushed by a Le Creuset, her neck decapitated by her old Ken Hom wok, her body, motionless, buried under a downpour of weighty cookware.

Mercifully, she was alive. Pushing away the debris surrounding her, I lifted her up on her knees and made her release the IKEA *Skänka* sauteuse she had been searching for. Then, for a moment, she rested quietly against me.

'Idiot,' I said, checking her skull for damage.

'I smashed the Gonal,' she sniffed, pointing into the collapsed culinary mountain. It was true; the Gonal had been taken out by a baking tray. A thorough search revealed only a single dose had survived the crash. A day's supply.

'Bugger,' Martha muttered to herself. Then she cooked hamburgers.

The following morning I headed off towards St William's. We both had work deadlines, but it was agreed Martha's was tougher; her first ever *Holby* script was due by five o'clock. I had a voice-over, but the recording didn't start until one. The day should have been straightforward, so it was a surprise when nine hours later Martha shouted at me:

'Do you really want this? Do you?' Her fist was trembling as I walked out the door.

The problems began as I weaved my way towards the hospital. I noticed Paxman trotting alongside me.

'They'll just die,' he said. 'Eventually your children, like you and Martha, will die and their children will die and what's the point of it all?'

'Shut up,' I snapped, walking faster.

'Imagine,' he continued, 'every day the fear for them – fear of disease, bullying, kidnap, broken limbs, perverts, and then the drinking, the smoking, the sex, marriage...'

Paxman paused. For effect.

'Then death,' he said. 'Always death.'

I stopped and turned to my one-time hero.

'Paxman,' I said, 'you're not helping.'

Paxman, surprised at this, disappeared. At the clinic the receptionist welcomed me with a new prescription and a scowl, and then sent me off to the hospital pharmacy.

It was located in a cavernous fluoro-lit hall in the centre of St William's. Row upon row of plastic chairs were bolted into the lino-tiled floor, uninhabited save for three old ladies, bunched together, waiting silently for something to happen.

In the far corner was a hatch and above it a sign read: The Pharmacy.

I migrated across to the hatch and peered through. Inside was a small cubicle with an unoccupied stool. I waited for a minute, then another. I noticed a button, like a doorbell, half-concealed under a slip of paper. I pressed it and somewhere, deep in the bowels of the hospital, a bell rang. Then nothing happened for a while longer.

I looked at my watch. 10.15.

Given adequate notice and resources, I have developed techniques to fight against my own impatience. A portable video game, a *What Pension?* magazine, codeine-based painkillers. Now I was naked. I had nothing but my work BlackBerry on me, and that only had Block Breaker, the worst game in the world; a game that made doing nothing into a game by comparison.

That's why BlackBerry got into trouble. If they'd installed Solitaire they would've been fine. That and not calling the parent company RIM.

'We're going to call ourselves RIM.'
 'RIM?'
 'Yep. From this day forward we're all going to be Rimmers.'
 'Really?'
 'What? You got a problem with rimming?'

An old man materialised. He sat down on the stool, adjusted some papers, looked confused at his own adjustments, and readjusted them again. Then, for reasons unknown, he gave his own head a little pat. Satisfied, his ancient eyes looked up and rested upon mine.

'Hi,' I said.

He responded with an almost imperceptible nod.

'I have this,' I pushed the prescription through the hatch.

He picked it up. It was as though he'd never seen a prescription before. Or paper. In fact his withered complexion suggested his first language might be Sanskrit, and that only some cruel accident of fate had set him down here rather than the British Museum. Gradually he deciphered the purpose of the strange papyrus in front of him. He placed it on top of the pile of papers and handed me a ticket. On it was printed the number '74'.

I looked around the waiting room. The three old women were all staring at a certain point to my left, their faces fixed in a state of paralysed boredom. I followed their gaze and discovered an electronic display on the wall.

It read '71'.

'When your number comes up,' the man said, speaking for the first time. 'Your prescription will be ready.'

'How long?' I asked.

He shrugged.

'Ten minutes?'

He shrugged. Our conversation had ended.

I looked at my watch. 10.24. How long could three numbers take? I sat down and pulled out my phone. The choice was either Rimmer's Block Breaker or staring at the display with the old women.

I sighed, clicked 'new game' and slumped into the seat.

Thirty minutes later I was still looking at the same number. Number 71. Not a single prescription had been issued for thirty minutes. What were they doing? Reinventing Gonal-f? Questing for fire?

The counter ticked over. Number 72 appeared. One of the pensioners, no doubt in her teens when she arrived, staggered towards the hatch. A swift twenty minutes later '73' came up. I clutched the ticket in my hands. I was going to make it!

Then it happened. Once again the display ticked over. My legs, coiled springs ready to propel me across the room, steeled themselves. My eyes widened, my throat dry. I looked up to the electronic sign, the herald of my exit from this place, my saviour...

... And there was the number. And the number was 75.

I glanced down at my ticket: 74. I blinked and looked up: 75.

Knocking the last of the old women out of the way, I threw myself at the hatch.

'Excuse me,' I said, my hands shaking with rage. 'You've missed my number.'

Ancient Man looked back at me. He let out a long, wheezing breath, possibly an evolutionary forerunner to the sigh.

'Which number?' he said.

'Which number? There's only been four in the past hour. You went from number seventy-three to number seventy-five, circumventing my number.'

He stared at me.

'Which number?' he repeated.

'Which number? The number that comes after seventy-three and before seventy-five. Surely you can count?'

He was a pharmacist. Counting must have come up at some stage. I pushed the ticket towards him.

'Number seventy-four. I'm number seventy-four.'

'I'm seventy-five,' an old woman's voice cried from behind. I shot her a look to let her know that if she ever wanted to see her precious seventy-five, she better wait. Quietly.

Instead she started to nudge me out of the way.

'Number seventy-five,' she cried again.

I nudged back, continuing to shout into the hatch.

'Where's number seventy-four?'

The man looked at his notes.

'Let me check, sometimes if we get an emergency...'

'People come to you in an emergency?'

'I'll just check,' he said, shuffling off.

'Number seventy-five,' the old lady cried, trying to push her ticket into the hatch. The man returned.

'We're out of it.'

'Out of what? Gonal-f? Time?'

'It won't be in until this afternoon.'

'This afternoon?'

'Yes.'

'I can't do this afternoon.'

'This afternoon,' he repeated.

'Bloody troglodyte,' I hissed, waving a fist at the man.

'Seventy-five!'

Outside, I thanked security for escorting me from the building and looked at my watch. I took a deep breath. I could do this. I had time; I would finish the voice-over by four, giving me an hour to get back to St William's, pick up the prescription, go home and stab Martha. It was going to be fine.

And it was until I arrived at post-production. Then I remembered who the voice-over artist was. I smiled and shook his hand, sat down in the dubbing suite, glanced over the script, and only then put my head into my hands and groaned. The sound engineer next to me nodded.

'Yep,' he said. 'We're doomed.'

We were doomed; we had booked the industry-renowned Mr Pedantry.

'So,' Pedantry said, five minutes into the script. 'Nauseous.'

'Sorry to hear that,' I replied, trying to insert sympathy into my voice.

'No,' he rubbed his chin, 'You've used the word 'nauseous' here.'

'Yes,' I replied. 'The character is nauseous.'

'Really?' Mr Pedantry's eyes glowed. 'The character has the ability to cause nausea?'

'No,' I said. 'He's nauseous. He's feeling sick.'

'Ahhh,' he nodded, crossing out the word. 'So he was nauseated then.'

Mr Pedantry was always just on the right side of wrong. Google was unable to completely disprove his incessant nit-picking regarding the correct adjective for an unpleasant sensation of the stomach, though the OED did come down on the side of the script. After several minutes' discussion, we finally all agreed that it would be safer not to risk using 'nauseous' and go with 'nauseated' instead.

'You see,' he smiled, tapping the side of his head. 'Useful for something.'

Not for the continuation of the human race, he wasn't. Sadly, it was not the only grammatical, historical or sociological ambiguity in the script. Each ill-placed comma or ambiguous reference required further reflection on the nature of language or being, and the pharmacy was well and truly shut by the time I arrived.

I was an angry man when I walked into our flat and announced there was to be no Gonal stab-fest that evening.

'Oh, genius,' Martha crossed her arms. 'Absolute genius. What are we going to do now?'

'It'll be fine,' I said and tried to explain about the nausea.

'Thanks,' Martha interrupted, having none of it, 'for putting our future family somewhere below poor grammar.'

'I didn't do it. Mr Pedantry did.'

'Well, it's nice to see you and Pedantry getting on so well.'

Martha was being cruel. I didn't have celebrity friends. I was the only TV producer in the world unable to form the dysfunctional bond required to be mates with a famous person.

'I don't care about Pedantry,' I snapped. 'Actually, I don't care about the drugs and I don't care about the baby. I don't care.'

Men sometimes say they don't care. Usually they say it just at the moment when they care the most, when the thing they care about is in desperate need of that care, and when admitting that they did care would sort everything out. Why Martha couldn't see that I don't know; instead we had a fight, which ended with her shouting: 'Do you really want this? Do you?'

I walked out. I stood outside our flat, surprised at the question, my heart beating fast and hard, but I couldn't tell whether it was rage or fear or both. Did I want it? Was something in me trying to jeopardise our baby-making efforts?

Suddenly my mouth went dry again. This time I could feel the dust on my tongue, hear a child crying; the back of my neck was warm as though the sun was on it. It was like, like...

Paxman stood next to me.

'What is it?' I asked.

'I think you'll find I do the questions,' he muttered and disappeared again.

The dryness passed. I went to meet my friend Rob – we had agreed weeks ago to a catch-up and off we went to The Bleeding Heart, a pub where young lovers mixed with groups of overweight drunken lawyers chatting up the barmaid. We edged our way to a corner table and sat down. Rob placed a fatherly hand on my shoulder.

'We'd like…' he paused to examine the colour of his wine. 'We'd love you and Martha to be godparents to our kids.'

I was shocked. Godparents. It was an honour. A privilege. A joy. So why did it feel like the last scrape at the absolute bottom of the parenting barrel.

'We'd love to!' I replied.

I felt a meta-guilt about feeling guilty about recoiling from this generous offer, but it occurred to me that this might be the closest we'd ever get to being parents. Godparents could be it. Godparents fall below the parents, the grandparents, the great-grandparents, the cousins, the half-siblings and that teacher they had who migrated to New Zealand and sent a postcard once.

No one ever takes a godparent seriously.

'Hi, we're the parents.'

'Well, we're the godparents. Beat that.'

'We do beat that.'

'Really?'

'Yes. Biologically, legally, emotionally and as a social construct, we are superior to you in all ways.'

Eventually, unable to hide in the pub any longer, I went home. All the lights had been turned off in the flat and I could hear Martha in the bedroom. She was doing her best pretending-to-be-asleep breathing. It never works – she can't even get her respiratory system to lie. I went in, not sure what to say, not sure whether to apologise or to argue or to beg.

'We're godparents,' I said, sitting at her side.

My eyes adjusted to the dark. Now I could see Martha, lying in the bed, looking up at me. Then I saw us on a Sunday morning, in a suburban street, waiting outside a freshly painted door in some not-too-distant future. We were holding a present between us, waiting for someone to come to the door. Inside, children and parents playing and laughing and alive. Outside, us and our present.

Then we were alone, in the middle of the party, still holding our unwanted gift, a little island isolated from the world by a sea of children.

Martha switched on the bedside light.

'This can't beat us,' she said. 'We need those drugs.'

I heard the front door close. It was Why leaving the flat.

I nodded. We'd lost precious days to this existentialist nonsense, having the crux of very existence undermined, but we had learned something. 'Why' was not a word for grown-ups cut off from the object of their desire. 'Why' wasn't for us; 'why' was for our future child, looking at clouds in the sky or wondering why dinosaurs don't eat chocolate, or whatever. 'Why' wasn't even for the baby we wanted.

'Why' was for the baby we needed.

'Masturbatum contra mundum?' Martha asked, putting her hand onto my chest.

'Masturbatum contra mundum,' I nodded, my hand moving over hers. Then I fell into bed. Then the alarm buzzed and I got up and went down to the pharmacy to do battle with The Troglodyte.

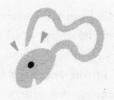

Chapter 11

Death of Sex

Time for a montage.

Martha doing sit-ups on the recently cleaned Xthorp rug. Me on the Internet. Martha jogging in a park. Me pulling my trousers down. Martha tossing a salad. Me staring at a girl's buttocks wiggling on the screen. Martha discovering me, trousers down, looking at buttocks. An argument. Me pointing at the screen, the buttocks being injected by a trained professional. Martha, understanding, massaging my shoulder while I practise stabbing myself. Various close-ups of me crying in pain.

Finally, Martha and I on the sofa, smiling, post-coital, looking contentedly at an empty syringe.

'It didn't hurt,' Martha hugging me like I'm Indiana Jones.

Then cut to me on a farm looking at a sheep. Someone hands me a satellite phone.

'It's your wife,' Harry, the director, said, sniggering.

I was annoyed with Harry. I understood that the greatest shepherds of Britain and Ireland, about to compete in that year's *One Man and His Dog,* were unimpressed with my new violet-gloss Hunters, but he didn't need to join in. He lived in Hackney.

'It's all they had left,' I protested, begging Harry to appreciate a sophisticated Wellington; but Harry had gone native and went back to more footwear jokes with the judges. To this day there are farmers out there, still laughing about the media-boy's purple wellies.

Gripping the bulky eighties-style handset, I began to walk up a muddy hill where someone had once got a signal. You would imagine we were somewhere exotic: Somalia, North Korea, the Urals; but no, those places all have a phone network. We were in the Lake District. Here even satellite coverage was patchy. You'd think the telecom companies would look at a map of the United Kingdom, feel shame, and realise that the object of a mobile network was fairly obvious, it being in the name.

I reached the pinnacle before Martha's voice finally crackled into life.

'I'm not pregnant,' she shouted over intergalactic interference. 'I'm not pregnant.'

Then a cloud or a bird or a Sontaran spaceship cut the signal. Martha had sounded different. Still upset, still disappointed, but determined. We had made a pact. We had decided to take control, to be the masters of our own fate.

I looked around: England, from up high, was a beautiful sight: green, peaceful and, above all, fertile. Out there everything – the sheep, the birds, the trees, the flowers, the grass, the fish – everything was reproducing without thinking about it. Everything except us.

Then I stepped on a dead lamb.

'Arse,' I muttered.

I walked down to further mirth at my bloodied footwear. Then it began to rain.

Two days later Martha and I faced the perfectly composed features of the undead Nurse Ratched. We had a plan. The original plan was based on Bram Stoker, but that was vetoed by Martha and English common law. The modified plan was this: go as hard as we could without killing anyone. St William's obsession with IUI stood in the way of us and IVF and the only way to rid ourselves of it was to push IUI harder than IUI had ever been pushed before.

'Up the dosage,' Martha said, her eyes upping the price of steel.

'I'm not sure,' Nurse Ratched replied. A porcelain finger came to her lower lip. 'Your ovulations seem normal.'

She was right. They could set atomic time using Martha's ovaries. Even I could tell she was healthy. The problem was elsewhere; perhaps my sperm were having trouble finding their way. This would come as no surprise – I often can't find things. Or ways. Up to now this had been an endearing quality, much loved by all those around me.

'Roo, have you seen my *Flightless Birds of the UK* book?' I might ask.

'It's on the table,' she would cry, trying to get dressed.

'What table?' I would ask, looking around for a table.

'The table,' she would answer.

Suddenly the table would appear in front of me. I would go to it and look. There would be no book on the table. Hard as my eyes searched, I could see nothing. My wife was wrong.

'It's not here,' I would cry back. There would be a pause, the sigh of lost hope from the other room, and then Martha would come and look at the table, then look at me, and then motion for me to look at the table once again.

On it would be the book. It was like magic. It was like things came in and out of existence depending on whether or not Martha was in the room.

So I imagined my sperm would fare poorly in the obstacle course of the female reproductive system.

'Hey, the eggnav isn't working.'

'Let's just say we got lost and hit the pub.'

'In this pink get-up? No fear – I'll just ask that antibody for directions.'

Back in the clinic, Nurse Ratched continued her resistance. She knew what we wanted: to prove, once and for all, whether conception could happen inside Martha by turbo-boosting her reproductive system. We were going to turn her ovaries up to 'eleven'.

'Up the dose,' Martha repeated.

'It could be risky,' Nurse Ratched shook her head.

Indeed. We might risk having a wanted pregnancy. I raised my index finger and pointed it at Ratched.

'Up the dose,' I said.

The dose was upped. We were going to give IUI another try, this time with a monstrous load of egg-inducing Gonal-f.

We also clung to the faint hope of conception the old-fashioned way: having actual sex. We had now arrived at the third stage of intimacy in a malfunctioning reproductive relationship and sex had become like a major infrastructure project or a Mormon's relationship status on Facebook: it was complicated.

Intercourse had once been simple. It worked like this:

'Sex?'

'Brilliant.'

Then sex.

Then came the second stage: scheduled sex arrived.

'Sex?'

'Scheduled or non-scheduled?'

Then sex.

Now sex required project management. Our month went like this: no sex for the three days before hospital foursome sex. Afterwards, a quick bout of scheduled sex. Then, sex in the shadow of imminent test results. Then, disappointment and bitterness at our own useless sexing. Then, on the seventh day of Martha's next cycle, at around 2.15 p.m., spontaneous sex.

'I'm in Cardiff,' I said, checking the diary.

'Stupid Welsh,' Martha muttered, as though they were responsible for our ills.

Trying for a baby had become like a weed. It was infecting every part of our intimate life and the new, powerful injections of Gonal-f were like manure. As the drug poured through Martha her body began to change.

I was a sensitive chap. I didn't want to embarrass my wife; she was going through enough. I thought I'd keep these new sensations to myself, wait for the right moment to bring it up.

'Something downstairs is weird,' I finally blurted out. Martha lifted her head slowly and turned to me.

'You want to talk about this now?' she whispered.

I looked up. To be fair, we were at a christening. We were sitting near the back of a little Victorian church in south London, listening to a priest go on about the importance of something to do with God and the baby. There were many truly awful hats. What happens to the heads of middle-aged women that they require such unattractive headgear?

'The drugs,' I said, 'are having side effects.'

Someone coughed. The priest sprinkled water on the baby's head.

'Ferning,' Martha sighed. Ferning? I considered the word. I looked around at our friends; they were all at the naming-ceremony stage in their lives. Some had even progressed from child to children. Some had finished making their families. We, on the other hand, had arrived at the mysterious 'ferning'.

The baby began to cry. It was not the right time to inquire further. 'Ferning' didn't sound like it was going to bring joy; in fact it sounded like something you might do with and/or to a shrub. Other signs also suggested I should leave 'ferning' well alone. For example, Darwin was now sitting on the pew next to me.

'Don't ask about the ferning,' he whispered.

'What's ferning?' I squeaked.

Martha stared at me. *Really?*

'Ferning,' she paused, covering her face with her hands, 'is the excessive production of cervical mucus.'

Darwin shook his head frantically. *Don't talk about the ferning!*

'Sorry?'

The priest muttered something about the devil.

'Cervical mucus,' she hissed through her palms. 'I have lots of cervical mucus.'

Cervical mucus. Could they not have found a different name for it? Nectar, for example. I might have been able to cope with, say, fertility nectar. That could have worked.

They wouldn't do it to men. They don't call sperm 'penal snot' or 'squelch', yet the nomenclature unit at the WHO or UNIT or whoever rules on these matters had somehow decided that mucus was a perfect descriptor for it.

'Why are we calling this cervical mucus?'

'It's got a catchy ring to it.'

'You're comparing vaginal lubrication to a runny nose.'

'Geez, you chicks get tetchy. What is it? Time of the month?'

I should've left it. Not gone any further. After all, where has curiosity got us? Killed, that's where. Look at that bloke in *The Evil Dead* – what did curiosity do for him?

'Don't go into the cellar. It never works out well.'

'But I'm curious.'

'Your girlfriend has just been molested by a tree and, to be frank, I don't think she was ferning at the time.'

I couldn't stop. Curiosity forced me to enter my own metaphorical *Evil Dead* cellar and discover the truth.

'But what is it?' I asked, shutting the trapdoor behind me.

'What's cervical mucus?'

'Yes!'

Outside the church, eager to avoid spending more time with another baby that wasn't ours, Martha took me to one side and explained: cervical mucus was an indicator of ovulation and that now she was being stimulated by the drugs, she was producing more of it.

'So it's helping us get pregnant?' I said, relieved. It was like oil in an engine. A working hyperdrive on the Millennium Falcon. I could see that. I could deal with that.

'Possibly,' Martha looked evasive.

'Possibly?'

'Well, I could have hostile cervical mucus...'

I nodded. Of course she could. Of course there was something called hostile cervical mucus. I glanced around – if only I could get my hands on Darwin for five seconds...

'... in which case it will actually trap and kill the sperm inside me.'

Hostile, sperm-killing, cervical mucus. The whole thing was vintage Star Trek. I couldn't imagine Captain James T. Kirk allowing angry vaginal phlegm to threaten his foxy young alien wenches.

'It's cervical mucus, Captain – if it gets any closer it might infect the hot she-babes of the planet Fertillium.'

'Set everything to "annihilate" and pack the K-Y.'

Martha was taking a drug that was potentially building an anti-fertility wall inside her. Surely we were now the only couple in the world whose reproductive treatment seemed designed to prevent conception at all costs. We sat down on a bench facing an old Victorian gravestone. It read:

Here lies Jeremy Flingo, beloved father and husband, lovingly remembered by his children Charles, Scarlett, Mary, Tobias, Anthony, Pearl, William, Sarah, George, James, Sebastian, Henry, and Myrtle.

'Oh, for Christ's sake,' I muttered. Even the dead were more fertile than us.

'Spinnbarkeit,' Martha slipped her arm through mine. 'Spinnbarkeit is the medical term.'

Spinnbarkeit. I could deal with spinnbarkeit. Don't tell me what it means. I don't want to know. For all you Germans out there, forget spinnbarkeit and use cervical mucus instead.

Martha's head rested on my shoulder. Suddenly, surrounded by the virile dead, a wave of optimism surged through me. After all, ferning was the best indicator that Martha was ovulating, and that it was going to be an ovulation of biblical proportions. Isn't that what we wanted? I looked up to the heavens and there was Jeremy Flingo looking down, in his morning suit, waving a fist as if to say:

'Go get 'em, tiger.'

Two days later Martha came home from a scan at the clinic.

'They think I'm overstimulated,' she said.

'Excellent,' I said, but something in Martha's voice suggested this was not in any way excellent.

'No,' she said. 'They think I'm really overstimulated. They want to see us.'

Suddenly we were in front of Nurse Ratched again.

'You're overstimulated.' She shook her head.

'Isn't that good?' I asked. Surely we wanted Martha's reproductive system stimulated?

Nurse Ratched showed us the ultrasound. She pointed to numerous clear white strands in Martha's ovary.

'Each of those is a follicle with an egg,' she said. 'Each of those is a potential baby.'

Martha's face dropped. I counted the white lines. Fifteen strands. Fifteen eggs.

'But this is good,' I insisted. 'Fifteen chances at a baby. How can that not be good?'

Nurse Ratched looked at me.

'It's not fifteen chances for a baby,' she said. 'If IUI was successful, your wife would almost certainly have a multiple pregnancy.'

'And?' So we might get twins. Get it all out of the way. Job done. I continued to stare at the fifteen lines.

'Not twins.' Nurse Ratched shook her head. 'Fifteen. Martha could produce anything up to fifteen embryos.'

I stared at her for a moment and then over at Martha. Her silence was enough. Was it even worth asking the question?

'We can't…?'

'Do you know what happens with this kind of multiple pregnancy?' An odd expression appeared on Nurse Ratched's face. Was it disappointment? Mild frustration?

I shook my head. Aliens?

'Nothing good, Mr Cossey, nothing good.' She then turned to Martha. I recognised the expression now. It was sympathy.

'We need to cancel this cycle of IUI,' she said softly. 'I'm sorry.'

Martha nodded, our grand strategy defeated.

We went outside. Martha had been supercharged for nothing. We had pushed her body to its limits and it had done everything asked of it. Inside, over a dozen eggs were waiting to be fertilised, a Jeremy Flingo-ful of potential Cosseys. All of them completely useless.

Later on, a cursory look at the Internet revealed the horrors of high multiples in pregnancy. Premature birth, defects, death. All the words you didn't want associated with reproduction. Martha bit her nails, her knee jogging up and down.

'It's our fault,' she said.

'Look…' I searched for something to console her. 'Let's go to a nice restaurant, have a meal, and then afterwards we can have traditional, unscheduled, fun sex.'

Martha's knee kept jogging. What had I done this time? I picked up my mobile to reserve a table.

'We can't.' She shook her head.

'Can't go to a restaurant?'

'Have sex! We can't have sex for the rest of the month because my ovaries are carrying a football team. With substitutes!'

I looked at my wife, uncomprehending.

'We,' she said, 'can no longer do it. Shag. Make love. Have relations. Nothing.'

Silence.

The truth of the situation finally dawned on me. Well, I thought. Well, well, well. Well. This was a step forward. This was true progress. We had started from infertility and, thanks to modern medicine, we had arrived at abstinence. We had come to the point where even bad, emotionally scarring sex was impossible.

Martha and I had been demoted to good chums.

And the reason intercourse was outlawed? Because it might lead to the very thing we most wanted: babies. The treatment now recommended by the St William's Centre for Reproductive Medicine was not to reproduce at all; not to have any kind of sexual contact, or in any other way allow conception to take place.

'A condom?' I suggested. How desperate was I, mentioning the plastic? The word I thought had ceased to exist, an object I had dismissed from my life.

'There's fifteen of them,' Martha cried.

That night, as I struggled to pull a second condom over my reluctant member, First Girlfriend appeared at the end of the bed:

'Two-condom Cossey,' she smiled, twirling a finger through her peroxide perm. I stared at her – surely my imagination was exaggerating the size of those shoulder pads?

'Go away,' I said, but she just shook her head slowly.

'I thought you'd be trying for a baby by now.'

'I am trying for a baby!' I shouted, snapping on condom number two.

It was no use. After twenty-three years of sexual activity Two-condom Cossey failed to live up to his name. I threw them to one side and lay on our marital bed with just my untouchable buddy-wife, my first girlfriend, and two barely used prophylactics for company.

I was angry. I searched around for someone to take it out on. The undead Nurse Ratched? But there was her face; kind, empathetic. She had warned us against our overstimulation folly. Suddenly a dozen puffins appeared on the bed, covering Martha. Each one seemed wounded in some way, a bandage around the head, a wing in a sling, a limp. Each one stared at me with a mournful cuteness.

'Club us', they seemed to say. Go on, for the baby, give us a good clubbing.

I looked at my Alan Border signed cricket bat, standing in the far corner of the room, but even for a baby I couldn't beat wounded puffins. With a collective sigh, they vanished.

It had been almost three years of the monthly cycle of hope followed by despair, and this month we'd taken a short cut around hope and gone straight to the despair bit. Later that night, I felt Martha's hand take mine and guide it to her belly. For a while she said nothing, just lay there, holding my palm above the multiple eggs growing inside.

'At this moment,' she whispered. 'I'd take a football team. I'd take anything.' I nodded. For reasons unknown we were being denied a baby, our sex life was in ruins, and as for the future?

IVF is not a guarantee...

Do you really want this? Do you?

'Can't they get rid of some of them?' I asked. 'Leave us with twins or something.'

'No, Roo,' Martha replied, lying still. 'They can't.'

I wanted Martha to have a baby. I wanted us to have a family. I didn't want to be lying here, next to a wife I couldn't make love to, waiting for a child that might never arrive. I wanted to be a father.

Or a wizard or an astronaut. I would take being an astronaut, though the current British space programme wasn't looking positive. Still, I could dream; dream of escaping above the earth, floating outside the international space station, watching over our little planet.

'You wouldn't like it,' Martha interrupted. 'Drifting above six billion people and knowing you hadn't produced a single one of them.'

She was right. I didn't want someone calling me a spaceman. I wanted someone to call me 'Dad'.

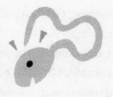

Chapter 12

Life's a Picnic

'Congratulations.' A portly chap called Neil took my hand and shook it.

It was the sixtieth birthday of a close family friend. Not one for doing things quietly, he assembled those closest to him one Sunday afternoon in October at a west London restaurant. Alongside his wife and children were aging cousins, siblings, nieces and nephews, friends from school, university, work; all there to celebrate a successful life as a father, a husband, and an all-round decent man.

'Thanks,' I replied, wondering what I was being lauded for. I took my place next to a spritely, silver-haired woman.

'So pleased to hear about Martha,' she muttered, reaching for the butter.

I smiled. Everyone seemed so positive about us all of a sudden.

'After all, she wasn't getting any younger,' she continued. 'And the things you hear these days.'

'What?'

'Women leaving it too late. Getting all dried up inside.'

'Sorry?' I asked.

'Creeps up on you, it does, creeps up on you.'

Unable to change a subject I didn't understand, I turned away from the crazed pensioner to discover congratulatory Neil sitting on my left. I waited for more praise, but his eyes were fixed on an event happening across the table.

Martha was drinking water.

It was not possible, on this day, in the sunny environs of west London, with numerous toasts and the chinking of crystal, that my wife would sit quietly nursing a glass of water.

The news spread quickly and the eyes of the party fell upon Martha's hand, once again lifting the symbolic H_2O towards her lips. Could something else be in the glass? Vodka? Had Martha, since the last gathering, become a hardened alcoholic? But no, nearby was a jug. You don't have a jug of vodka – the only thing you have in a jug is water, and where there is water, there is life.

'Not drinking?' smiled her neighbour.

Martha, suddenly aware of the expectant silence around her, hurriedly put the glass down, but it was too late: the effort of months hiding behind alcohol-free cocktails and secret orders of tonic water had been for nothing. With a single sip, Martha had provided diehard proof of her own pregnancy, because the only reason to drink the stuff was a baby, a religious conversion, or imminent liver failure.

And Martha wasn't yellow.

What no one understood was that water was also, confusingly, diehard proof of fertility treatment. Martha was purifying her body.

People winked at me, nudged me, initiated me into the world of the parent.

'Family,' nodded Neil, his arm falling over my shoulder. 'It's all about family.'

What was this, *EastEnders*? Before the Mitchells and the Watts it wasn't always about family and, even if it was, everyone didn't go on about it. Also, if family was so important, why was everyone in Walford always forgetting their surname? Every episode it's 'I'm a Mitchell' or 'Remember, you're a Branning' and so on.

'Family,' Neil repeated, pulling me closer.

'What does that actually mean?' I asked.

'Not sure.' He considered the concept for a minute. 'I'm divorced anyway. The kids live in Watford.'

It was now clear that, for the purposes of lunch, Martha was pregnant. Biologically she might have been as barren as the moon, but socially we were mere months from having our own bouncing little Anaximander or Ramses.

'Oh, you know the sex then?'

Someone nodded.

On the way home, Martha glared at me.

'Anaximander?' she said.

'What's wrong with that?' I laughed. Everyone else seemed to be naming their babies after obscure Roman generals; I was just riffing back to the Presocratics.

Martha got out of the cab.

'What are we doing?' I asked.

'It's not funny,' she said as I paid off the driver. 'There are forty people back there who now think I'm up the duff with

187

an Ancient Greek philosopher. By tomorrow that'll turn into a hundred. There'll be cards in the post soon.'

I shrugged. People were idiots and there was nothing to be done.

'It's humiliating,' Martha said. 'Don't you understand how humiliating it is?'

I shrugged again. People were...

'Shut up,' she snapped. 'Anaxi-bloody-mander.'

Martha and I were not getting on brilliantly. Nowhere was this more apparent than back at the clinic where she remained silent while I argued with the Ratched.

'We're not doing it,' I said firmly.

Undead Nurse Ratched shrugged.

'Don't shrug at me,' I shouted.

'You seem frustrated.'

'Thanks, Zombie Freud. I am frustrated.'

'Mark!' Martha gave me a look.

'Just IVF my wife,' I raised my hands to the heavens. 'Go on. Just once.'

'We need to see if a lower dose of the Gonal-f can...'

'Can do what?' I stood up. 'Help her ovulate? She ovulates. She one hundred and ten per cent ovulates. If there was a show called *Strictly Come Ovulating*, she would win it.'

Nurse Ratched crossed her legs.

'Mr Cossey, sit down.'

'We're not doing it,' I repeated, sitting down. I dropped my hand, waiting for Martha's to meet it, but it wasn't there. She was looking at the floor, biting her nails.

'Hello?' I asked, slightly annoyed. Was I now fighting the forces of darkness on my own?

Later, back at home, Martha showed me an email.

From: Sarah Morgan
To: Martha
Hi Guys
Long time no see! We're having a little picnic for the twins' second birthday (I know, I know time passes quickly for everyone except us!) – we'd love you to come and celebrate it...

'We're not doing that either,' I muttered.

Two hours later I was stabbing Martha on the sofa. We were, apparently, doing it. It was now dawning on us that our lack of fertility was in fact a chronic condition. It could go on indefinitely, forever being treated, forever in a sort of reproductive limbo. It was like emotional diabetes.

'We need to come out,' Martha said. 'We need to tell people.'

Turned out we had been outed long ago. Fertility treatment had long overtaken television as the most routine thing in our lives, and we worked in television, went to the pub with other people who worked in television, then came home and watched television. So it shouldn't have been a surprise that all humanity already knew about the subfertile Cossey household.

'I knew you were firing blanks,' said a work friend.

'Really?'

'Yeah,' he laughed. 'You told HR. What an idiot.'

Stupid HR. Everyone knew that if you wanted to keep a secret at work you went to the publicity department.

Now I felt humiliated. Suddenly I could see the subtle behavioural changes which had built up around us. The look in every parent's eyes as we approached them: *don't mention the kids, don't mention the kids.* We were lepers. Or their kids were lepers and the parents were also lepers and they were trying to protect us as the last non-lepers of humanity. Anyway, there was definitely a leper thing going on. People desperately creating child-free zones around us. Whispered conversations in the kitchens: 'Keep them away from the sterile Cosseys.'

Yet even within this baby-and-toddler-free zone, there was no escape. We shared less and less in common with our be-childed brethren.

Take poo. Every new parent I met would, without fail and within five minutes, bring up the word 'poo'. If there was more than one parent they would begin a competitive poo discussion as to whose offspring could produce the most amazing faeces. The criteria for success varied: it could be volume or frequency or, in one specific case, distance travelled.

How could I contribute to such conversations? Could I talk about my own numerous, bowel-centric concerns?

'I could talk about your poo,' I suggested to Martha.

'Nope.' Martha gave me a stern look. 'Why don't you just invent someone with bowel problems?'

I came up with Billy The Fudge – a 1920s prohibition gangster – and then Martha told me to shut up and that we were going to see some childless people for a change. We needed a break.

'But who?' I asked.

'Single Mike,' Martha replied.

Of course. Single Mike. Good old perpetually single, sexually ambiguous Mike. Our sex life might be up the spout, our friendships reduced to an embarrassed charity, but at least we could still go to a dinner party and get drunk and talk politics until the early hours. We could park our troubles for at least one evening.

Mike greeted us at his front door.

'Friends.' He scooped us into his arms. 'How terrible for you.' Eh?

'Simply awful,' he said, trapping us in a warm, sweaty embrace. How can people still have body odour in the twenty-first century? How? It's called deodorant and it's available everywhere.

'Still, hope springs…' Martha attempted a muffled reply.

'Brave, so brave.' He rocked us gently.

We struggled helplessly as Mike dragged us inside, continuing to lament our shared woe. In fact, Mike appeared more upset about our fertility problems than we were.

He had also shared this pain with the rest of the assembled guests. Inside, we were confronted by the collective expression of a group welcoming survivors from a Russian Gulag for canapés. Tearful, Michael placed us next to a puffy-eyed woman whose dress appeared to be made from hessian. She reeked of jasmine and patchouli.

'Have you tried alternatives?' Hessian Woman asked immediately, leaning towards us.

'Have you tried clothes?' I replied, but only in my head. I think it was only in my head. It's never clear.

'Alternatives?' Martha asked.

'You now, acupuncture, hypno, diet. I know a wonderful herbalist…'

My heart sank to the bottom of the Mariana Trench, dug a hole, took out a harpoon gun, and shot itself. The futility of going public with our problem was now laid out before me. If everyone knew that we knew that they knew, everyone could advise. Be a critic. A confidant. Anyone could share their own road-to-conception map with us. The key thing now was to not engage with any of it. I gave Martha the clear signal not to engage.

'You know something about alternative medicine?' Martha asked, engaging. Why did she do that? Why did she never listen to me? Why did she always engage? If she was in the army there wouldn't be a United Kingdom left.

'What have you done?'
'I've engaged, sir.'
'You've bombed China. Again.'

Thanks to Martha's compulsive engagement disorder, we were herded into a conversational ghetto with a vegan muppet.

'I do know a bit…' The woman replied. I screamed internally. Knowing 'a bit' is the most harmful force in the universe, especially when it's applied. The guys at Chernobyl knew 'a bit' about nuclear energy, the captain of the *Titanic* knew 'a bit' about icebergs. Martha knows 'a bit' about ice skating and we don't talk of that day on the rink anymore; we just don't go skating. It's for the best.

Hessian Woman listed the kind of remedies that might be of use: fertility brews of nettles, dong quai and raspberry leaves, wolfberry supplements, sesame oil enemas (because everything is more effective when stuck up your arse), hypnotherapy.

On she went, critiquing western medicine for all its failings.

'Do you know what the word antibiotic means?' she said to me.

'No,' I moaned, staring at a candle. Was hessian flammable?

'Anti-life. Anti-life.' She shook her head. 'You see?'

I did not. What I saw was death from boredom unless she stopped reeling off the locations of meditation retreats in Scotland, yabbering on endlessly about the one thing we didn't want to talk about. When we got home I added her to the list of things to be burned on the arrival of our baby. What a special day that would be.

'Our sex life is dead,' I said, slumping into our sofa.

Martha nodded.

'Our social life is dead,' I said.

Martha nodded.

'What next?'

It didn't take long. I was brushing my teeth when I noticed it; a whiff of something in the air. I went into the kitchen.

'Is that sesame?' I asked, pointing my toothbrush accusingly at my wife. Martha looked sheepish.

'Can't hurt, can it?' she said.

It can. The anal cavity is a sensitive place. During my university days I'd worked as a porter in a hospital and men would occasionally turn up with something up their rectum. It never panned out. There was always an excuse for the object's location but none for the forty-eight hours it had taken them to get help.

If you do find yourself in this position, don't fret. Do not spend two days constipated trying to concoct an excuse. No one will believe you. There's no jury in A&E looking for reasonable doubt. Everyone knows what you did, and providing your choice of object was original – past successes include the humble light bulb and a marsupial – you're actually doing them a favour. They'll dine out on it for years.

'It's not a light bulb,' Martha said. 'It's an enema. It might help us get pregnant.'

I looked at my wife – heard the desperate desire to try something, anything to increase our chances of conception. Had it come to this?

'I'm not doing it, Roo.' I shook my head.

'I'm not asking you to,' she replied, but she was. I took hold of her and placed her bottom firmly on the sofa.

'Boo,' I said, putting a hand on each thigh and pressing down. 'I'm happy to inject proper medicines, prescribed by proper doctors, into your arse. I'm happy to wank into a jar and have my sperm turned into a colour last seen in a *Meg and Mog* book. I'll do pretty much anything, but I'm not sticking cooking oil from East Asia up your rectum because some useless hippy said it might help.'

Martha nodded.

'Horny goat weed?' she suggested.

'No horny goats up your arse either!'

'It's taken orally,' Martha pleaded. I paused. I looked at her, just to be clear we both knew what orally meant.

Martha rolled her eyes. 'I'm not the one who gets confused about the word "oral".'

I rubbed my cheeks. We had always scoffed at alternative medicine; at needles being stuck in your neck and strange herbs being rubbed on your crotch and whatever other quackery the world had devised to part infertile fools from their money. But that was before, years before. Now, as desperation sank in, horny goats seemed almost reasonable.

'All right,' I agreed. 'We'll do the goats. It won't work, but let's do it.'

Was I right? Perhaps the goats would do the trick; perhaps acupuncture and diet and the odd enema or two would flick a switch in the ecosystem of our bodies. I saw a herd of horny farm animals chasing my sperm down Martha's uterus.

'We've gotta get to those eggs before they do!' Sperm Number One screams.

'Too late, too late...' cries Sperm Number Two as a randy cow charges past.

A month later I was back in the wankatorium, full of supplements, trying to remember what an erection was and how to achieve it. Then the phone rang.

'Dad,' I said.

'We're outside your door,' he chirped.

'Dad...'

'I've knocked several times.'

'Dad, I'm in the hospital,' I whispered. Only my father could somehow synchronise his arrival from Australia to coincide with Martha's ovulation, and then completely forget we would be incommunicado when he landed.

'Are you ill?'

'No...'

'The queues at Heathrow were awful.'

'Dad, can you just call Martha?'

'Why would I call Martha?'

'Because I'm trying to... I just...' There really was no good way to explain medically assisted reproduction to a parent. Talking him through my current predicament would be like explaining basic economic theory to the Greeks.

'I'll call you back,' I said.

'Battery's a bit low.'

'You've been on a plane for twenty-four hours. How can your battery be low?'

'We'll just wait until you get back.'

'No, Dad...' He hung up. I called Martha in reception.

'Hi.'

'Hi. Shouldn't you be, you know...?'

'Dad just rang.'

'What?'

'They're outside the flat.'

'Did you tell them we were busy?'

'Can you just go and let them in?'

Martha hung up and went home to let my parents into the flat.

'British Airways was terrible,' my father announced.

Martha rushed back. This time, instead of whales mating, some kind of pan-pipe music was playing.

'Why can't you get some proper tunes?' I asked the nurse.

'Copyright.'

'What?'

'You need a licence to play commercial music. Anyway, this is a good pan-pipe mix. We find it helps people relax.'

I didn't need my sperm to be relaxed. I needed them to get off their collective arses and find Martha's egg. I needed Elgar's 'Nimrod', followed by 'Eye of the Tiger' and Chumbawamba.

We arrived back at the flat to find my father waiting, watching daytime TV. My stepmother had gone to check into the hotel. Martha put the kettle on and went into the bedroom.

I considered the old man next to me. We were never the world's greatest communicators. The combination of being men, being Australian, and having socially dysfunctional careers like mathematician and TV producer was never going to create an *Oprah* moment. Still, if ever there was a moment to connect, it was now.

I sat down next to him, not sure where to begin. Where did I start? How did I explain pink sperm and overstimulation to a man, near seventy, who used to take me to the cricket even though he didn't like it, who once dived into a river to rescue my sister from a water snake?

'Dad,' I said. 'We're having problems having a baby.'

Dad looked at me, his eyes bloodshot through his glasses, his beard grey.

'Mark,' he said, without hesitation, his voice soft. 'Martha's a good woman. It'll be fine.'

Then he sat back to watch the TV.

'Unlike British Airways,' he frowned. 'They were terrible.'

The only people left to tell were the Morgans. On the morning of the twins' party Martha was sitting in our bedroom, pulling on a dress.

'Going somewhere?' I asked.

'They want us to come,' Martha pushed her hair in several directions, unable to decide what was best. 'It's important to them.'

'Roo, it's a baby picnic.'

I hated picnics. I don't have the knees for them. It rains. Everything gets too warm and there's nothing to do and you can't escape and the food is unstructured and people try and make you drink Chilean Chardonnay. It's disgusting. Add babies to the mix and there is a fair chance it will kill us.

'We'll go for an hour, I'll get a headache, we'll go home,' Martha softened her voice. 'It'll be OK.'

We arrived at the back yard of the Morgans. Directly in front of us was a man, pinning his toddler child down, pushing a finger into its mouth. Above him the mother shouted:

'Get it out, get it out!'

Watching were three other toddlers, a little unsteady on their feet, wondering what all the fuss was about. One of them, a girl, chewed on a worm.

Martha and I glanced at each other. Hands held firmly, in we went. We ducked and dived through the mass of humanity. All around us were the conversations of parenthood, endlessly recycled.

'Five o'clock – every morning this week – we think it's the pox – three days before they cut her open – no, blanching's when the colour doesn't come back – and this poo, you should've seen it, we had to cut her out of...'

Suddenly an upside-down female crotch in a leotard appeared in front of us. It took us a moment to identify the object in its odd context and then, embarrassed by having stared at it for longer than was probably acceptable, Martha looked up and I down. There I discovered the owner of the crotch peering up at me, a fairy skirt hanging around her breasts, her yellow hair gelled into a sort of arrowhead. She gave me a brief smile and then cartwheeled off deeper into the throng.

We found our host, at the centre of the chaos, handing out drinks.

'Hey,' Sarah smiled, hugging Martha. 'Glad you made it. Mad, isn't it?'

I nodded in agreement. Troy and his toddler friends – Venus, Octavian, and Augustus – were screaming happily at each other.

'So?' Sarah asked. 'How's life?'

Martha bit her lip. Something flickered across her face but the smile held. Then someone handed her a baby called Maximus. I knew Maximus; he was what is technically known as an evil baby, and he began to retch a little on Martha's top.

'Actually, we're having fertility treatment,' Martha admitted, trying to give the baby back, but the mother had disappeared.

Sarah nodded. 'We'd guessed.'

'Really?'

'Yeah,' she said. 'I think most people have.'

There was nothing else to say. The three of us looked around at the dozen or so children; walking, playing, some saying their first words. It dawned on me how much further on in life people were. Even if Martha got pregnant now, the Morgan's kids would be almost three years ahead of us. Three years.

'Sorry,' Sarah apologised for the scene. 'I just want to keep things normal for you. Whatever that is.'

Maximus vomited with more force, covering Martha in milky sickness. She froze.

'Max!' Sarah cried.

'It's OK,' Martha said, putting Maximus down on the rug. It was obvious now there was something wrong with her, something beyond the puking baby, but I couldn't put my finger on it. I began to close in on my wife.

Maximus started to cry. The mother, her back turned, now heard the unique wail of her firstborn. She swung around to find her offspring abandoned on the ground.

'You could've just given him back,' the mother snapped, scooping up her son.

'I…' Martha stumbled, sick dripping off her.

'You,' said the mother pulling Maximus to her bosom, 'don't know about children, do you?'

A switch flicked. Twice in my life I have seen it; that sudden change in Martha, when murder comes into her eyes. This time it burned, bright and furious, met the woman's gaze, and unleashed hell.

'Fuck you,' Martha said, a 'fuck you' of such cold force that it cut through the toddlers' and the parents' chat and the cartwheeling crotch.

'Fuck you,' she said again, taking a single step toward Maximus and his mother. Then the rage fell away and Martha put a hand to her mouth, defeated.

'Come on,' Sarah took Martha's arm and started to pull her inside. 'Come on, let's get you cleaned up.'

We retreated. The mother, in shock, looked for her husband. Maximus, his work done, smiled contentedly. We passed Steve, staring at us, an unopened bottle of beer in his hand. The crotch started to move again. Kids named Eleanor, Beatrice, Herb, Frank and Otto chased after it.

Then we were outside, fleeing from the picnic. Then the truth came out.

'I'm bleeding.' Martha stopped.

'What?' It was too early. Too early in her cycle by days. Martha walked with quick steps down the high street, her face contorted, followed by the smell of baby sick.

You don't know about babies, do you?

'Fuck her,' Martha said, but the power in her voice had gone.

We got home. She went to have a bath, to hide away. I took her clothes and pushed them into the washing machine.

'This,' I said to myself, 'won't do.'

Then my mouth went dry. Again I could feel the dust on my tongue, down my throat, up my nose. I could hear the crying, see light at the edge of the darkness. I was almost there, wherever there was.

'Gravel,' I whispered. I was tasting gravel. But why?

Then it passed. I stood up. We couldn't go on like this. There had to be some kind of end, however bad it was going to be.

Later, with Martha safely tucked up in bed, I went on the Internet. I knew what I was looking for, but it was still hard to find. The number was hidden deep within the St William's website, obscured by false trails and difficult terminology, but eventually it yielded.

I rang PALS. They were people employed by the hospital to take the patient's side, to help you navigate the bureaucracy of the NHS. A woman answered the phone; I explained how we couldn't go back. Couldn't talk to Nurse Ratched or see Geoffrey anymore. How pointless IUI was, how no one listened.

The humiliation of my wife.

'OK,' the woman said. 'Let me help.'

Help. It was the first time anyone had said the word. A simple, powerful word that doesn't get said enough. Help.

And she did. A week later we sat in front of the Italian consultant.

'You want to give up on IUI?' he said, crestfallen. I had to give them credit. IUI was like a god to them. No amount of evidence to the contrary would convince them that IUI couldn't get a rabbit pregnant. We stared back at him, the evil stare of the unrequited parent-to-be.

'Puffins,' I said.

'What?'

The consultant stared at me. I smiled. He returned to our notes.

'You know the next step?'

We did. The Lamborghini of assisted pregnancy. The Michelangelo of up-the-duffing, of child creation.

IVF. Finally, IVF.

The consultant put down his medical rationing book and sighed.

'Right, we better get you booked in...'

Outside the clinic we stood for a moment, side by side, facing the world. The whistle had blown. Finally, we were going over the top, elated and frightened at the same time, and there was no turning back. I was almost forty, Martha well into her thirties.

If IVF failed?

Summer was on its way; we were another step closer to a life with, or without, children.

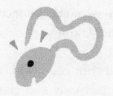

Chapter 13

Back to School

What no one told us was that a course *of* IVF also meant a course *on* IVF. Treatment kicked off in a theatre – a lecture theatre. Martha and I began our final confrontation with infertility not in a hospital, not in a consultation room, but by going back to school. Weeks before the first needle went in a letter arrived in the post, inviting us to a compulsory seminar.

'How can we be invited to something that's compulsory?' I asked. Where were we, Russia?

'We're going,' Martha said, poking me. Then, surprised by something, she poked me again, this time in the belly.

'Are you losing weight?' she asked.

'No,' I said, feeling my midriff.

Martha poked me again.

'Don't you want to know how IVF works?'

I knew enough. I knew IVF involved an intrusive operation which required my wife to be sedated. This, I thought, was brilliant news. They don't operate unless they're serious about fixing you up. That's why the most terrifying word in the English language is 'inoperable'.

'Mr Cossey, I'm afraid your condition is inoperable.'
    'Oh well, all those incisions and clamps did look painful. What's the alternative? A syrup?'
    'Well, no…'

'Any more details than "it's an operation"?' Martha interrupted.
    Details? When did the patient bother with details? I assumed someone would give us a brief explanation which we would ignore, get us to sign a form we wouldn't read, and then get on with cutting my wife open and putting some kind of baby in her.
    Instead we had to go to a seminar. What other medical procedure has a seminar? Everything else is just 'straightforward' with 'a small risk', and then suddenly you're in the foetal position with your trousers around your ankles.

'They're going to stick that up my what?'
    'You signed the form.'
    'It's six feet long!'
    'Well, your bowels are actually…'

Medicine would rather you didn't know what a rectal biopsy or amputation of the orchids means until it's too late. Otherwise you wouldn't go.
    Except fertility. Here there is a genuine, heartfelt attempt to put you off the whole thing. The Portakabins, the pink sperm, the anti-wank chair. The naming conventions of the

female lubrication system; it's an all-out attempt to stop you wasting everybody's time with your snivelling little fecundity issues. There is simply no other treatment where you need to be taught it before you take it. Can you imagine?

'I've got brain cancer.'

'Right, let's get you on the "Brain Cancer and Me" course...'

'It's quite aggressive brain cancer.'

'Exactly – you need to do the course before you forget everything.'

Martha gave up poking me. I doubted she wanted to go to a lecture on IVF any more than I did. In fact she probably wanted it less: the whole thing was just part of the continual, low-level embarrassment you were required to feel as a member of the subfertile race.

I stood up.

'Where are you going?' Martha asked.

'Sharpen my pencils,' I said.

If they wanted to send two liberal arts students back to school, then we'd show them what we were made of.

It is an unfortunate fact that the last time I'd studied science was when I mistakenly signed up for first-year Chemistry at university. I was asked to leave after I set the laboratory on fire. I know what you're thinking, Two-condom Cossey and all that, but it wasn't my fault. I owned the only box of matches in the room and the ventilation in the fume cupboard wasn't working. Our lecturer – who walked funny because he'd edged backwards off a mountain while studying rocks – decided that a room full of young adults, some carcinogens, and a lot of flammable reagents was a great place to fire up the new Bunsen burners.

'… and then,' I opened my arms, another fascinating story of my youth narrated, 'they told me not to come back. Me.'

I looked around, but Martha had disappeared.

IVF enrolment day arrived. Alongside us were several other couples, a few women with other women, and one guy on his own. Not sure what that was all about.

I glanced around at my fellow infertile freshmen and women. They all had pads out on their little desks. Martha, the competitive streak coming out, had assembled her own arsenal of stationery: fibre-tipped pens, pencils, an eraser, three notepads and, of course, Post-it notes in multiple colours. I myself had gone minimalist: a single notebook, a biro, and a box of matches just in case.

A young-looking woman entered the hall. She was smartly dressed, carrying a laptop which she deftly hooked up to an overhead projector. She clicked quickly through several carefully prepared PowerPoint slides, each full of bullet points and flow charts and diagrams of reproductive organs. Satisfied with her materials, she returned to the front of the hall and introduced herself:

'Hi, I'm Sam and I'm one of the embryologists at the clinic. Over the next hour or so, I'm going to talk you through the process involved in completing a round of IVF.'

An hour? How complicated was this going to be?

'It is complicated,' she continued. 'Especially compared to previous treatments many of you've been on. You may want to take notes.'

Everyone readied their biros to do hard labour on foolscap. Then I noticed something about my hand – it was blue. I had a blue hand. Was I bleeding? Why was my blood blue?

'Your pen's leaking,' Martha noted without looking up.

I was penless. I turned to my loving wife for help but no; she was already focused on the first slide, her fibre-tip furiously at work. Academically, I was on my own; I was going to have to concentrate, try and remember what was being said. *Focus*, I whispered to myself, *focus*.

'Now,' Sam brought up the first slide, 'today we're going to look at what we call the long protocol…'

Protocol? There was a word I wasn't expecting. Protocol is more your action man/diplomat kind of word. Protocols were the sorts of things that James Bond would ignore.

'… the long protocol in often used in women who…'

I wondered how 007 would take to IVF. More to the point, who would he do it – IVF, that is – with? He obviously had some kind of problem, shagging all those women and not one of them turning up on the doorstep a few years later, sullen little sprog in hand, shouting: 'Don't give me that old "you've got to save the world from the Russians" – we agreed Tuesdays and every second weekend…'

Maybe he'd have IVF with Miss Moneypenny:

'Did you follow the protocols, James?'

'I most certainly did not, but Pussy Galore did help me obtain a sample.'

Enter Q to collect Bond's generously filled jar of blue-coloured sperm.

'What are you going to do with that?' Bond says, raising an eyebrow to the camera. But we all knew what Q was going to do with Bond's sperm. He was going to shake it, but not...

'Now the overall timescale for the cycle you'll be doing is roughly three months...'

The embryologist's voice pulled me back into the room. Three months? How could it take three bloody months? It wouldn't take Q three months. All they had to do was get Martha's eggs out, dollop a little sperm on them, wait for one to start growing, and then pop it back in. Three months?

'... to take control of the woman's reproductive system we medically induce the menopause...'

Bond vanished instantly. Menopause? The menopause? The thing that stops women having babies in perpetuity? I needed to concentrate. I looked around; everyone else was happily jotting down MENOPAUSE in their notebooks. As though the menopause was a big plus for a couple wanting a baby.

Then there was something about overstimulation and some agricultural terms started to appear, with talk of what constituted a good harvest. I knew about farming from my time as a producer on *One Man and His Dog*, but what was the connection?

'Arr, where's young Timmy?'

'Arr, he be out fetching the menopausal sheep for the harvesting.'

'Arr. Come-bye, Timmy, come-bye...'

Photographs of different-sized embryos appeared, each graded from A to E, with A being excellent and E meaning your baby would grow up to be the bass player in New Zealand's second-best Iron Maiden tribute band.

The lecture ended. Sam took a few questions, which were all along the lines of 'what are my chances?' For the first time it became obvious that many in the group had real medical problems. Unlike us, whatever wasn't working in their reproductive systems had been diagnosed.

I did feel for them. They had all come here, taken notes, seen the effort involved, and not blinked despite their far-diminished chance of conception. Here were couples who were willing to go through years of invasive, difficult treatment with only the smallest hope that one day they might hold their own flesh and blood.

On the other hand, at least they knew the score. We had no idea. There was either some undiscovered fault in our physical make-up or we were just incredibly unlucky.

Then came the forms. One seemed very important; it asked us what we would like to happen to any remaining embryos and whether we would allow their use in research or not. I studied the question:

'If you do not want your embryos not to be used in medical research, do not tick the box marked "I do not give my consent."'

After much deliberation, I realised the quadruple negative had defeated me and ticked a box at random. This ensured that our surviving embryos were either saved for further use or sold to the American government for gene-splicing with the Roswell alien. Another document appeared. This one was asking me for a thousand pounds to store our embryos for future use.

'A grand?'

'It's for storage of our potential future children,' said Martha.

'A thousand pounds to freeze a couple of embryos. They're only the size of pinheads.'

'They're nothing like the size of pinheads. They're microscopic.'

'Unlike the price,' I cried. 'It's astronomical!'

I chortled. Martha and the rest of the room failed to follow my lead. It was hard sometimes to understand why Martha didn't appreciate my punning, but I guess she was about to go through the menopause. I ticked the box, agreeing to store any embryos for five years in case they were needed. Then we all shuffled out of the room silently towards the hospital pharmacy to wait dutifully for our drugs.

It was like an anti-freshers week, where everyone desperately didn't want to get to know each other. As we waited for a fresh batch of stabbing fluid to be brewed up in The Troglodyte's cauldron, I glanced around at my infertile compatriots. It occurred to me that during this whole process Martha and I had never really considered our fellow sufferers.

I had expected the men in the group to be thinking along the same lines. We would catch each other's eye, nod imperceptibly in recognition of the fact that we had actually caught each other's eye, followed by the faintest hint of a smile as if to tell each other 'we have caught each other's eyes, and nodded imperceptibly'. Then, one of us would pointedly pull out some phone or other recently acquired gadget, and the other, seeing the all-clear signal given, would nudge an inch closer, examine the device, and say:

'Is that the latest thingy?'

'It's actually the latest thingy plus,' would come the correct reply. An appreciative nod of the head was all that was then required for contact to be made.

This bond established, we would then communicate in typical male fashion.

'First cycle?'

'Yep. You?'

'Yep.'

Pause.

'Well, see you round.'

'Yep.'

But here, in the limbo of the pharmacy, no one caught my eye. Partners looked at the floor, or at their ticket, or just off into the distance. Anywhere but the eyes of their fellow man.

It struck me: we would never talk to each other. We couldn't. We were all in transition, but it was not clear yet which destination we were going to. Some people in the room were climbing up to the purgatory of crying babies, dirty nappies and sleepless nights; others to the hell of 'hobbies' and breaking into puffin sanctuaries with a crowbar.

None of us could strike up an acquaintance, a friendship, because at any moment one of us might be lucky, the other not. It was too fundamental a thing. We were all the walking dead; stuck between getting the most important gift in the world, and getting nothing.

And judgement day was inching closer. The quest for a child was no longer an infinite horizon with possibilities stretching out endlessly into the future, but a diminishing number of 'cycles' which, if unsuccessful, left only quackery and hope in the fertility arsenal.

We were near the beginning or the end, but it wasn't clear which. I sat down next to Martha, the blood draining from my face.

'You OK?' she said, looking up from May's *Kitchen and Bathroom* magazine.

'Fine,' was all I could think to say, but it wasn't. It wasn't fine at all.

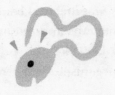

Chapter 14

A Brief Perimenopause in the Fabric of Time

It was a Thursday evening. Sunny, warm with a cooling breeze, the weekend in sight. People laughed in pubs, bathed in the golden rays that flooded London's parks, and somewhere, someone was firing up the first barbecue of the year.

It was on a spring day like this that I pulled out the big needle marked:

'Warning: contains the menopause'.

I approached Martha with gentle steps. I was apprehensive, unsure, frightened; throughout my life the media had been brutally honest about what was about to happen to my wife.

We were going to play god, nay the devil, with her hormones. I was Dr Frankenstein, hoping to create life with a single injection, but in reality about to bring a monster into existence. An alien. A demon. Not a good-natured sort like Mork or

Hellboy, but a thing of pure wickedness. A thing like the thing in the movie which was appropriately called *The Thing*. A creature which looked like you or me, but underneath was a life-sucking organism bent on the destruction of humanity.

That was the menopause.

Hot flushes, swollen ankles, terrifying mood swings. Insomnia, itchy skin, loss of vaginal elasticity. That clearly wasn't good. I was about to polymorph my wife into the Creature from the Black Lagoon, complete with inelastic sexual organs.

I had no choice but to confront Martha about this imminent change in our lives.

'This menopause thing.'

'Yep.'

'You're not going to go nuts, are you?'

'What?'

Of course I understood why we were doing it and that it was much worse for her. Still, after three and a half years of failed procreation, the last thing I needed was an early-onset menopausal madwoman stalking around the flat.

'Just remember,' I said, holding up the needle, bidding my wife farewell, 'I love you.'

'It's not a chemical execution,' Martha snapped. 'We're just halting my reproductive system for a bit.'

Because that's the way to have a baby, I thought – take out the principal baby-making machine by neutering it. I wondered whether we weren't part of some secret anti-baby experiment. Maybe MI6 was trying to outdo the Chinese.

'Let's go for a no-baby policy. That'll show them who's in charge.'

I injected the drug into Martha. Then I stared into her eyes, looking for 'the change'. I waited. Nothing happened. I waited some more, but her face didn't turn red and her ankles didn't swell. There was no foaming at the mouth or unusual growls. It was almost a disappointment. Had the drugs not worked? Where was the menopause? I looked back into her eyes, searching...

'Stop it now,' Martha pushed me away. 'It's not going to be that bad.'

It was. The following day I came home from work to find Martha sitting on our sofa, silently staring out the window. A single finger toyed with her hair and she was humming 'Somewhere Over the Rainbow'. A candle flickered on the table. The smell of peppermint wafted through the air and there was something else, something I couldn't quite put my finger on, a word I could only half-remember.

Peace. Our flat was peaceful.

It was all wrong. Terribly wrong. Our flat is never peaceful. Martha never sits silently staring out the window. She doesn't hum in a contented manner. She sings 'Teenage Dirtbag' in public places and swears at cyclists. They deserve it of course: always coming onto the bloody pavement and shouting at pedestrians who somehow fail to see them hurtling along in their silent, unlit, almost invisible two-wheeled machines of death, but Martha sometimes went too far. She once accosted

Boris Johnson about London's plethora of two-wheeled maniacs. While he was cycling. On the pavement.

Most importantly, my wife never ever does nothing. Her days are full of lists, productivity, and the occasional piece of amateur detective work.

Now she was lounging. *Lounging*. Just staring out at the buildings on the other side of our road.

'Roo?' I said quietly, cautiously sitting down next to her.

'Mmm?'

'You OK?'

There was a long pause.

'Just relaxing.'

'Relaxing?'

'Relaxing. Have you ever looked out the window and thought, well, not thought anything?'

No. I look out the window and think why are they digging up the road again? It's been dug up a dozen times already; what else could possibly lie beneath it? Elvis? The lost city of Atlantis? Why don't they fit everything into some kind of underground pipe and then send a trained monkey down when something goes wrong? And why can't they do it quietly? How can we precision-attack an al-Qaeda headquarters in the remote hills of Pakistan with something called a Stealth Bomber, but not fix a leaky water pipe without forty different types of digger turning up, each with their own special ear-splitting sound effect?

'Bumpkin,' Martha trailed a finger down my arm. 'They're just doing their job. Digging up stuff.'

Bumpkin? When did bumpkin happen?

'Are those cupcakes?' I cried, staring at a plate on our sorry-looking Xthorp rug.

I wondered whether Martha needed a hospital. A special hospital. Had it all gotten too much – had my wife finally cracked? Had she been given the wrong drug? Had I unwittingly injected her with some kind of slow-acting opiate whose side effects included baking?

Over the next few minutes I did my best to break the spell. I threatened to invite annoying friends over, quote from the works of Alain de Botton, go double denim by wearing jeans with a matching jacket, but nothing seemed to work. Motivated Martha had turned into Methadone Martha.

'Look,' I said, opening a centre-page spread in some women's supplement. 'Here's an article about how women make men more gay.'

'Coolio,' she replied, making the peace sign with her hand. I couldn't stand it anymore. She had been this way for five minutes.

'What is wrong with you?' I asked.

'Wrong?'

'You're wearing sandals.'

'It's the menopause, Roo,' she said dreamily, standing up and doing a pirouette across the living room.

This was the menopause? I shuddered. What was next? Glastonbury? I didn't want to go to a music festival with my hippified wife. I didn't want to go and sit in mud and listen to distorted guitars playing songs I'd never heard of while thirty-somethings lost their Platinum Visa cards rutting each other in a muddy tent.

What had those monsters done to her?

'But the menopause,' I objected, pouring peppermint tea down the sink, 'is all about women going mad and complaining about room temperature.'

Martha scanned our limited CD collection.

'Actually, that's the perimenopause.'

Perimenopause? What was that? Portuguese for a bleeding chicken? A side order at Nando's?

'The perimenopause is the bit when your body goes through the change,' she said, inserting a CD into our stereo. 'Menopause is technically the bit after. And it's rather pleasant.'

She turned to me. 'Don't you just love Kate Bush?'

'No, I like Bryan Adams and other good Canadian artists,' I said, wanting my old wife back. It was like being in Huxley's *Brave New World*, except with 'Wuthering Heights' playing in the background.

Still, I thought, at least at the end of this they would IVF her and then we might have our baby.

The following morning, as our spiritual journey through the menopause continued, the pigeons arrived. Something in our balcony flowerpots had attracted them. Was it the wilting flowers? The olive tree which somehow wasn't alive but wouldn't die? The broken stump of a bush I planted last summer?

For a moment it wasn't clear and I ignored their squawks as I concentrated on de-menopausing the flat. I tried bear-baiting Martha by reading out what Gordon Brown was saying. I do feel sorry for the bloke; his parents had the last name Brown and then they stumped for Gordon. You're never going to get the lead in the school play with a name like that.

'We need someone with character, with gravitas, with passion!'

'What about young Anthony Blair?'

'Of course. Let him take the lead in *Whamlet*, our Shakespeare musical set to the tunes of George Michael.'

'And Gordon?'

'Props.'

It was not until this strategy failed to get Martha off the couch that I noticed a small pile of twigs, dirt and bird shit being assembled underneath the remains of the bush. Next to it stood one of the pigeons. I stared at it; it stared back at me with an innocent, nothing-to-see-here kind of look.

Something was going on and I called Martha over. I waited the several minutes it now took her to float across the living room.

'They're building a nest,' she said.

I looked again at the randomly assembled bird grotto in front of me. That shapeless pile of twigs covered in white pigeon poo was a nest? Pigeons really were disgusting creatures, I thought, rightly hated by all good Londoners.

'I'll get the bat,' I nodded. The air-rats could find somewhere else to raise their harpy brood.

'No.' Martha raised a chilled-out, menopaused hand. 'Maybe it's a sign.'

A sign? It was now obvious we had been somehow teleported to Middle-earth and Martha had become a slightly unhinged elf-wench from Rivendell. For an instant I felt slightly frisky.

'A sign of what?' I asked. 'Infectious disease? Your mental health?'

'Please.' Martha placed her hand over mine and looked lovingly at me, then carried that loving gaze down to the pigeon. I don't think the pigeon had ever been looked at with love before. It clucked nervously. Then daddy pigeon turned up with a plastic sugar-stirrer in his beak.

'It is a sign, Roo,' Martha confirmed with a ponderous nod. 'It's like your puffin thing. Love them like your puffins.'

'No, I don't...' I started and then stopped. Now was not the time to explain the puffins.

'A sign.' Martha floated off to make salad.

Signs. Signs are like the film *Signs*. Always a disappointment. A group of aliens disguised as frog-puppets invade earth only to discover they're allergic to water. Really? You've got intergalactic space flight, superweapons and the like, but you can't muster a defence against anyone with a tap. How, for example, were they planning to invade Manchester?

Yet, I thought, if festering-evil winged rodents reproducing on our balcony gave my menopausal wife hope, then who was I to object. The pigeons stayed.

With Martha now fully zoned out and our chances of getting pregnant once again reduced to less than zero, we did some socialising. Again we found ourselves at Single Mike's door. Here we were at least guaranteed some sort of epicurean pleasure.

'Poor people,' he cried, ushering us in. 'You poor, poor people...'

To be honest, Mike was more Martha's friend.

'We all need to get through this,' he sniffed, casting our jackets onto his bed. He was right. We, my wife and I, needed to get through this. He just had to get through dinner.

'I've got a tissue somewhere,' said Martha, messing around in her bag. I stared at her. Why was she giving Mike tissues for our problem? Where were my tissues?

I think Mike fancied her slightly, because while Martha got to sit between him and someone who sounded emotionally grounded, I ended up next to a man in his early thirties, dressed in a double-breasted pinstriped suit.

He seemed rather cold. I tried cricket, politics, TV, books and dogging as conversational openers. It always works when I talk about dogging. My parlance in outdoor spectator sex is both witty and post-modern, but he didn't laugh once. Everything was brutally brushed off with a shrug until finally he turned and looked directly at me.

'IVF,' he said. 'I don't believe in IVF.'

Mike would need tissues for more than tears in a moment, I thought. What did this gentleman mean? Did he mean he didn't believe in the actual existence of the medical treatment known as *in vitro* fertilisation? I agreed with him there – from the bits I understood it all sounded a bit far-fetched.

'That's not what I mean,' he raised both eyebrows. 'I mean it's a sin. A grave sin.'

Again I agreed. There were certainly some sinful aspects to the whole thing. The size of the jar, the endless injections, the pan pipes...

'NO!' he roared, dipping his unleavened bread into a bowl of Moroccan humus. 'It's a sin against God.'

Oh... I thought ... *dear!* He stared into my eyes. 'What about all those embryos that don't make it? What about their souls? In a few days you'll be a murderer.'

On he went. Apparently, because the IVF procedure doesn't always use all the embryos, and embryos are all human beings with souls, IVF is murder. Not to mention that this murder is committed by someone who had already committed the mortal sin of masturbation. I was about to become a murderous wanker and the man knew it.

'What do you say to that?' he finished, now stabbing a giant Malaysian tiger prawn with a fork and sticking it in his mouth.

I didn't know. I didn't want an embryo, I wanted a baby. A baby that would grow up, eat pizza, buy a house and have more babies. Embryo-destruction seemed a price worth paying. Embryos are being knocked off inside wombs around the world all the time. In natural conception it's estimated anything from twenty to seventy-five per cent of embryos just don't make it. It was also tricky to identify with something that only had eight cells and was microscopic.

'Get out much?'

No answer, because it's a microscopic organism.

'Doing anything interesting?'

Still no answer, because it's still a microscopic organism.

'Listen, I've paid five thousand quid for you and raised you since you were a single-celled nothing…'

I wanted to explain that nothing in nature suggested we should treat embryos as anything but potential human beings, but what was the point? I wanted to explain that we wanted to create life, not destroy it. We wanted a family and science just wanted to give us a little hand in achieving our aim.

I now know that, when you have problems, when you are feeling low in the uncertain struggle to create your own family, when the medically induced sterilisation of your partner seems a fair and reasonable thing to do, there are people who will hate you for it. They will have no problems expressing it. Once, at work, a colleague, on hearing that the NHS was paying for our treatment, snapped at me in anger.

'It's none of my business,' she said, 'but I don't see why my taxes should pay for your baby.'

'It is a medical condition,' I replied.

'Pfff. There are too many children in the world.'

No. There are too many children in countries with no family planning. This follows the little-known Cossey rule No. 2, which states that the poorer you are, the more the civilised world will force you to have children you can't afford; and the richer you are, the more it will try and stop you having the children you can afford. Rule No. 1 involves not leaving the diaphragm on the side table, and then hoping it will still work as form of contraception, but that's another story.

Back at Mike's, bread and bone marrow appeared on the table. The man, satisfied that he had put me in my appropriate plane of hell to rot for eternity, took a piece and dipped it into the gelatinous goo, raising it to his mouth.

I wondered what we should talk about next. Then it came to me.

'Ferning,' I said. 'Let me tell you about ferning...'

The menopause passed. Martha returned to her normal unsterilised self and we left our Huxley-based dystopia for the more Orwellian universe of Gonal-f and friends. Low-level criminal teenagers up to no good once again learned to fear my wife; who was that strange invisible vigilante that kept reporting them to the police for upsetting a flower tub?

Having shown such power in halting Martha's reproductive systems, the clinic invited us back to begin the reproductive reboot.

'So the menopause went smoothly,' Nurse Ratched said, tapping away at her keyboard. Why she brought it up was anyone's guess. No one was questioning St William's ability to put the brakes on conception. If they were looking to win a gold medal for the world's most expensive and unwanted birth control, it was theirs for the taking.

No, what we needed was the other bit. The bit where Martha got pregnant.

'So we'll start with ovarian overstimulation...' Nurse Ratched continued.

'We will not!' I stood up. I'd had enough. Bloody medical staff, didn't they realise what happened last time Martha became dangerously overstimulated? The return of Two-condom Cossey – that's what happened!

Martha covered her face with her hands. Behind her stood First Girlfriend, now dressed in a tasselled white leather jacket, her hair straightened and gelled. She waved a two-pack of Durex at me.

'Mr Cossey.' Ratched motioned for me to sit down. 'This time we *want* to overstimulate your wife.'

First Girlfriend vanished in the puff of an eighties smoke machine. I looked at Martha. She nodded, indicating that this time we did want to overstimulate.

'Did you both miss the seminar?' She began clicking on her mouse. 'I think there's another on Thursday.'

'We'll be fine.' Martha shook her head.

We arrived home to find our other family, the pigeons, had given birth. No problems with their fecundity then. While the nest was now a squalid rubbish tip, the birth had been anticipated as a continuation of 'the sign'. I'd imagined sweet, cottony-white chicks, crying out for their mother who would lovingly bring them food. I'd seen us watching them grow from fluffy cuteness into fully fledged pigeons, foreshadowing the arrival of our own offspring.

Of course, the problem with using pigeons as a metaphor was that their offspring looked like mutant rat foetuses with small beaks welded onto their mouths. And they sounded like rat foetuses who'd just had a beak welded to their mouths. There is the reason why pigeon chicks don't feature prominently in the rich tapestry of the western literary tradition.

'It's still a sign,' said Martha, slightly less convinced than before.

'A sign of what?' I wondered. Even the mother seemed confused, wondering what she had mated with to produce such an unpleasant trio of miniature gargoyles.

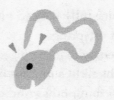

Chapter 15

Casualties

'What about some spare needles and medicine then?' I asked.

A shake of the head.

'Do you want my mobile number?'

'Not bothered,' the receptionist said, eyeing up a chocolate finger biscuit.

The big moment was drawing near. Soon Martha would have her final scan and, if that went well, someone from the hospital would call, giving us a date and time to come in for the egg retrieval. Then, precisely thirty-six hours before that, we had to pull out a further big, special needle and inject it into Martha.

If we failed to do this, if something went wrong, if we spilled the medicine or missed the phone call, then the whole thing was off and it would be another three-month wait.

This is why I wanted backup, just in case there was a Marthalanche or a terrorist attack or a small black hole appeared, sucking the trigger medicine into an alternative universe.

'Everyone else manages it,' the receptionist growled, continuing to look longingly at the finger.

CASUALTIES

I came home to find Martha and her mum sitting around the table.

'Everything OK?' I asked.

'All OK,' the thumbs went up. The thumbs were one of the seven signs that something had gone drastically wrong. The other six also involved Martha and her mother sitting around a table.

'What's up?'

Martha paused, then confessed:

'They think the trigger shot will be Wednesday now,' she admitted.

'You mean Thursday.'

'Wednesday.'

It had to be Thursday. Everything had been set up for Thursday. I had rearranged filming, edits and the laws of the universe to make Thursday work, all based on the empirical fact that Martha's ovulations were the atomic clock of the reproductive world.

'I'm away on Wednesday,' I said.

'You are away on Wednesday,' Martha confirmed. I would be trapped in a small town somewhere two hours from London. 'But don't worry,' she continued, 'Mum's going to do the trigger shot.'

I looked at Martha's mum.

'I basically work at a hospital,' her mum smiled.

'You teach ethics to medical students.'

'It'll be fine.'

I loved Martha. I loved her mum. The two of them and a needle was never going to work.

'I'll get out of it,' I said.

Up until now, except for the logistics of a juggled life between the great world cities of London, Los Angeles and – no prejudice – Cardiff, my job had never seriously conflicted with our treatment, so I expected sympathy.

'Work,' I now pleaded with my boss, 'is getting in the way of me stabbing my wife.'

'We've all got domestic issues,' he said miserably. 'You can stab her in your own time.'

What was so pressing, you ask? A live TV broadcast? The Director General's leaving video? Sadly no, it was the upcoming annual awayday and, more pertinently, whether or not my attendance was required. I was for not attending. My boss, however, was strongly for.

I don't know why. These things are torture. It's unlawful to detain people against their will, but, for reasons known only to the United Nations, the conventions on human rights do not apply to awaydays. According to work, the only place in existence where co-workers can bond is in a hotel somewhere up the M4. What kind of a bond they're hoping for is unclear: the Stockholm syndrome?

A compromise was agreed. I would attend on the Tuesday, do the first session on Wednesday and then get a train home, hopefully in time to inject the trigger shot.

The collective might of our department dragged itself into some dreary conference room. There the torture began with the 'sessions'. The ones where you get to 'know each other'. For what purpose? I already knew everyone; if I wanted to know them better I could just walk across the office and say 'hi'. I could have tea, an affair, go postal. Anything but an awayday.

In the first session an attempt was made to unlock our inner creativity. This was not a good idea; creativity is to the BBC what God is to the Church of England. Best not talked about. Best just let everyone get on as they see fit and not tie ourselves up in horrible knots about the whole thing.

Without the word 'creativity', no one would have to sit there listening to a 'guru'. Ours was a curly-haired, middle-aged man in a striped short-sleeved shirt, full of anecdotes, mainly involving something to do with a prostitute and an airline, which would unlock our inner muse. The question, never answered, was if his technique was so foolproof, why was he stuck talking to us and not out there being the next Michelangelo or inventing a replacement for the Angry Birds game?

Anyway, none of us wanted to unlock our inner muse. We weren't Buddhists, we worked in television – our inner muse had left us for a Brighton-based folk singer years ago. No one wanted to be there. We wanted to be in an edit, pontificating at some poor producer about whatever random thing was going on in our head while a series of images passed in front of us on a screen. This is known in the business as 'creative leadership'.

Next came the strategy session. A very nice lady from Audience Planning shocked us with the fact that TV audiences wanted to watch creative and engaging television that was new and fresh. Sadly, the truth is, no, they don't. They want the Doctor to save the universe, Clarkson to drive fast, and Ian Beale's head to be shoved down a toilet, before finishing the evening with Paxman giving it to someone with a halberd.

Eventually everyone went to a bad restaurant, ate awful food with people they once had feelings for before the awayday had destroyed all emotional will. Then I got an eye infection and went back to the hotel. I dreamt about the fertility clinic's awayday.

'Right, so how's objective "A building with foundations" going?'
  'We're still in a Portakabin.'
  'And operation "IUI – It Works!"?'
  'It doesn't.'
  'Well, have we got anyone pregnant then?'
  'Mary's cat had kittens...
  'Well, that's something.'
  '... they died.'
  Pause
  'Anyone for dinner, I booked us in at the Filthy Monkey...'

The next morning I went, as agreed, to my last session. There we all sat, half the department hung-over, the other half wishing they were, virtual guns at our heads, ready to blow our virtual brains out.

'Hey,' the session host clapped his hands. 'This year we're all going to tell each other an embarrassing story from our childhood.'

I had to stay for this? I considered my options – the most expedient answer was obvious. All I needed to say was:

'Something happened to me. As a child.'

Then add something about a special doll, burst into tears and leave. No one would make me go on an awayday ever again.

Too cowardly to imply some kind of childhood abuse, I confined myself to retelling the soft-toy massacre of my childhood. As I mimed a toy bunny being hung from the ceiling, everyone fell silent. Then I made my excuses and went home to stab my wife.

Three hours later, Martha rubbed her leg and looked up at me.

'Right then,' she said. 'We're on.'

We were on.

Two days later, out of respect for tradition, I pulled on one of my old pairs of loose boxer shorts. The colour had faded and there was a rip down one side, but even given their state they seemed looser than when I had first worn them.

I noticed The Gremlin sitting next to me. His trip to Thailand with Marv had clearly been hard on the little fellow; he looked tired, his hair grey in places, his back a little bowed. I noticed he had also donned a pair of old boxers. He stood up and saluted me. The pants fell to the floor.

I smiled and returned the salute. This was it. The moment of reckoning, of truth. With 'Jerusalem' playing in the background, I went off to the clinic to initiate what I now called the short-wank protocol.

Martha followed an hour later. This time we were ushered into the ward, the inner sanctum of the infertile. The final line of attack in the war for a baby. Martha changed into her theatre gown, got into the bed, and from there we studied our fellow hopefuls. Many of the women had already been through the procedure, had their eggs harvested, and were sleeping off the sedative. Some were sitting up quietly, reading a magazine while their partners sat, patiently, looking around for a nurse, wondering how it had all come to this.

No doubt someone, somewhere in this room, was already on their way to greeting their little Egon into the world.

'We're not calling it Egon.' Martha flipped through the July edition of *Kitchen and Bathroom*. 'Where do you get these names from?'

Ghostbusters and other top eighties films, obviously. I started humming the 'Ghostbusters' tune. 'I ain't 'fraid of no ghost. Dun dun dun na na na naaaa na. I ain't 'fraid of no ghost...'

People looked at me. I apologised for not being afraid of no ghost and sat down next to my wife.

The place didn't feel like a steaming hot laboratory of life, and it wasn't. No one in the room was in any way pregnant. The action all happened elsewhere; the introduction of my sperm to Martha's eggs would take place in a laboratory we'd never see. If all went well, some stranger would be the first one to witness the union of my sperm and her egg, our potential future son or daughter. A stranger who we'd never know, the kind of stranger who decided a career playing with sperm was a good option.

'Dad, I'm going to work with jizz.'

'Please, what about drug addiction? Have you thought about becoming a crack whore?'

'I just can't stop thinking about it. It's like a calling.'

'Join the Socialist Workers Party. Then you can hang around with wankers all the time...'

This was the kind of semen-loving man or woman who would see our potential newborn a good forty-eight hours before we did.

Martha's hands shook slightly, her eyes darting around the room.

'It'll be OK,' I said. 'We're on our way now.'

'I know,' she nodded. 'It's just the pain. You know how I am.'

I did know. Martha wasn't scared of the pain. She was frightened of the same thing we'd been terrified of since the beginning: the truth. Of finding out the answer to the one question we needed to know but didn't want to: could we have a baby? After IVF, there was nothing else, nothing stronger that the medical world could offer us. IVF was it.

For better or worse, the truth was coming.

'Roo,' I said, but that was as far as I got. There was nothing else to say. I became aware of just how powerless I was, what little more I could do.

The nurse and a porter appeared, put Martha onto a trolley, and took her away to have her eggs harvested. I sat down to wait.

I thought about our wedding night, how much had happened since, how much hadn't. I thought about the future, my desperation for us to have our own little family. Was it too much to ask?

I looked around at my fellow sufferers. Why were all these people, wanting to share their love to carry on the human race, denied it? What if IVF didn't work? What if we stayed childless forever? It was a near certainty that someone in that ward that day was never going to hold their own child. *Dear God*, I said by way of a selfish shameful prayer, *don't let it be us.*

Don't let it be us.

Martha returned, dozy and nauseous (or 'nauseated', or 'queasy', or 'not well in the stomach', or whatever). She drifted slowly back into the conscious world, smiled, then vomited. Then she wanted to know: how did it go? Then she wanted chocolate. Then she vomited again. Finally a nurse came out and told us: seven eggs. They had retrieved seven eggs.

'Are they good eggs?' Martha croaked. The nurse shrugged. We wouldn't know for another twenty-four hours.

It was the hardest day's wait. Up until that moment, no one knew the answer to that most basic question: could we conceive? Could we make an embryo, the first little step to creating a human being? I'd always believed that conception had never taken place, that my mischievous sperm had just never found Martha's eggs, that our problems were navigational. Now darker thoughts crossed my mind: could the quality of her eggs be poor? Could they just be rejecting my sperm?

That night and the next morning, we moved around like half-zombies, waiting for the embryologist to call and let us know whether we were still alive or not.

We tried to distract ourselves by heading down to the beach, as though some light surf and an ice cream might take our minds off it. Of course, nothing could take our minds off it. Being in a plane crash wouldn't take your mind off it.

'It's looking bad, Captain, real bad. Air pressure's gone, that thingy that keeps us stable...'
  'You mean the wing?'
  'That's it – well, it's fallen off I think...'
  'Bloody hell... oh, hang on, this call might be important...'

Martha's phone rang. She had a brief conversation with the embryologist, then hung up and held the phone tightly between her legs.

'Well?' I asked.

'Two grade As, the rest Bs.' Martha gave a pained little smile. 'He said we were top of the subfertile class!'

Top of the subfertile class! In your face, first-year chemistry. It was the best you could hope for. Never mind that the whole ranking system sounded slightly made up, never mind that I had no idea what being an A-grader did for your chances. We were the best and so were our embryos and, sweetest of all, we now knew we could conceive. Conceive! That meant Martha could get pregnant and that was the best news we had had in years. Everything was possible. We could have a baby.

'We could have twins,' I said.

Martha, ever fearful of the god Hubris, bit her lip and said nothing, but inside I could see something I hadn't seen for years. Inside her was hope: here was proof that we weren't infertile. In less than forty-eight hours Martha could be carrying our first child.

When we got home we went onto the balcony to reflect. I looked down at mother pigeon and her brood of festering rat-children. Maybe they were a sign after all. Then the monstrosities screeched at us until we retreated.

'They're growing up,' Martha said, slipping an arm around me. Even I, despite the fearful, unhealthy and disgusting mess that was now strewn across our balcony, felt a kinship with the little avian family in front of us. Sure, the area around them looked like the morning after a Tippex convention, but maybe Martha was right; maybe those mutant flying rodents were a beacon of hope; maybe we were going to have a baby.

Two days later we returned to transfer the embryos from the laboratory into Martha. We went back to the same old procedure room we had been to many times before. The pan pipes belted out unknown composition after unknown composition.

Geoffrey the embryologist explained that both the little grade As were doing good business, each of them now an eight-cell microscopic leviathan, ready to get growing inside Martha. I was becoming more and more convinced this was going to work. We were there. Good old IVF had sorted us out and now we just needed one of those embryos to take hold. Come on Cosseys!

The transfer completed, we went home. I studied my wife, looking for something that might indicate a change. I felt her belly.

'Feel pregnant yet?' I asked, putting an ear to her womb.

Martha put down her book.

'Boo,' she said. 'I think that's my liver.'

'Do you feel different though?'

But there was no answer. The next day I got up and went to work as normal. I sat down at my desk. I felt anxious but optimistic.

Then the phone rang.

'It's David,' Martha said, deadpan. Seconds passed. 'He's dead.'

'David's what?'

'He's dead.'

David was a university friend of Martha's, a lawyer, a decent guy. He was young, recently married, healthy, strong, sociable.

How could he be dead?

'OK,' I said, now hearing the shock in Martha's voice. A ruthless selfish streak came over me. I pushed David out of my mind. The one thing to do now was to keep Martha calm, to not let whatever had happened affect her or the potential baby growing inside her.

'He's been killed,' she said.

Killed?

'OK,' I repeated. 'Just stay calm.' There was nothing else to say. I turned around and went home.

It soon became clear that he had died violently. Everyone was in shock. It was unbelievable that such a thing could happen; we had cheered him at his thirtieth. I had missed his wedding because of a filming trip in Australia. At home I tried to talk Martha down, but it was impossible.

'I can't help feeling upset,' she said.

'OK,' I said, standing above her. 'But try and keep calm. Try not to think about it.'

Martha looked up at me. Was I so heartless?

'I can't help it,' she said and left the room.

I went down to the supermarket to buy some ready meals. London felt different; the sirens more menacing, harsher. I passed the reception of one city building and David's picture was on a giant screen. I thought of poor Ailsa, his wife, her life turned upside down by something so pointless. Then I felt selfish for thinking anything at all, because it was all just a distraction from my own terror, my own little drama that was now playing out. Soon Martha would do the test and we would know.

That night, for the first time ever, my beautiful wife lay beside me, not talking, not asking for anything, not moving. For the first time, we went to sleep without saying goodnight.

Nine days later it was the funeral. It was as David would have wanted, in his old college, a big audience there to remember him. The world came to celebrate his short time on this earth, and to steady and support those left behind. To witness the fact a life had passed by, too quickly, but was still remembered and known to all.

I was queuing for tea when Martha tugged my jacket.

'We need to go,' she said.

'We just got here.' I was surprised. A moment ago she had been hugging friends.

'We need to go. *Now.*'

We left. We walked down the path and back out of the college, and turned towards the station. Then, after we had put a hundred yards between us and the wake, Martha stopped. She sat down on a bench at a bus stop.

'I'm bleeding,' she said.

Tears ran down her face. I felt the warmth of summer. I looked up at the spires of an old church, then my gaze fell and watched a cyclist ride by on the cobbled road. Then I looked at the laces on my shoes and then a small crack in the concrete.

Years, I thought. Months, weeks and days, hours and minutes, all to arrive at this second in our lives. Scans, injections, operations, the menopause; two grade A embryos – our two potential little children – the best embryos in the world going into a perfectly healthy uterus. All of that so I could stand here and Martha could sit there, at a bus stop, bleeding.

I opened my hands. I wondered where my rage was. Where my desire to fight back, to scream against the unfairness of it all, had gone. Instead I tasted gravel. Gravel in my mouth, my throat, the inside of my cheeks. It was only when we squeezed into our seats on the crowded train home that it hit me. A memory from almost thirty years ago.

I was twelve. I was at my mother's funeral. I knew how important it was to be brave, to be quiet and listen to the priest and the other speakers and not cry, but I couldn't. I couldn't stop the tears. I ran out of the room and into the car park and threw myself at the gravel and begged God to change what had happened, to bring my mother home. Then I buried my face in the gravel, trying to block out the light, the pain, the unbearable loss.

Then the guilt. The guilt that I couldn't stay and say goodbye to her. Death had beaten me.

Now, again, I pushed myself into the dirt. Life had beaten me. We were never going to have a baby. I knew it in the core of my being. Never. I had failed and the price was losing everything, a family, Martha. The future.

As the train came into London I caught a glimpse of us, the Cosseys, reflected in one of the windows. We were thin, hollowed-out creatures with sunken eyes. We had become the thing I had mocked so long ago.

We were the new Skeletors.

PART 3

TRY HARD WITH A VENGEANCE

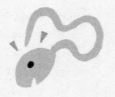

Chapter 16

First Girlfriend

First Girlfriend was pushing a lubricated cable down my throat. It was this, the near darkness of the room and the heaviness of my own body which made me suspect one of three things:

I had died and gone to hell.

The *Matrix* films were true.

First Girlfriend was giving me an endoscopy.

'Try not to gag,' she smiled, funnelling the cable in further. Her perm had disappeared and in its place was a heavily jelled, golden-coloured sculpture made from what was once hair; it clashed heavily with the reddened cheeks and glitter-covered lips.

In the shadows behind her I noticed The Gremlin, smoking a hookah pipe. Next to him an Italian, wearing a codpiece and a red robe, was scribbling notes. A strange screen in front of me broadcast meaningless black and white pictures. Somewhere in the background 'Just Can't Get Enough' by Depeche Mode was playing.

'Ahm hrying,' I replied. Then I gagged, my body trying to rid itself of the tubing. First Girlfriend paused, leaned down, and stared into my eyes.

'Are you all right, Mr Cossey?' she asked.

I considered the question. I reflected that, on balance, I was not.

After the failure of IVF and the funeral, Martha and I had arrived home to our empty nest. This is not a literary cliché: on top of everything the pigeon family had chosen that week to depart. Their nest stood abandoned save for one of the offspring, which lay buried under a half-hidden branch, lifeless.

I looked at Martha, but she was in no state to clean up dead pigeon. Some logic of marriage dictated this was man's work.

I snapped on a pair of plastic washing-up gloves and edged out onto the balcony with the bleach and a black bin liner. I waved a fist at the dead body of the half-grown bird in front of me. Martha had been right – the pigeons were a sign, their meaning now obvious. They were not some mystical fertility metaphor, not some indicator of future progeny. They were just life, our life; a messy old bric-a-brac of crap and broken eggshells.

I picked up the pigeon and pushed it into the liner. Then I attempted to yank the entangled sore of a nest from the earth, but its foundations were surprisingly sound. As I tugged harder, various voices went through my head: *IVF is not a guarantee. Do you really want it, do you? You don't know much about babies, do you? I'm bleeding. I'm bleeding. Negative. Negative. Negative…*

'What is this, Macbeth?' I shouted at my own brain, and then the nest suddenly surrendered. Large chunks of it splattered over the windows, the balcony, me. Bits of the disgusting rotting pigeon crap hit my arms, my chest, my face.

I went back inside.

'We need to get away,' I said.

'Escape our woes,' Martha nodded in agreement.

Then I was gagging again.

'This'll be a little uncomfortable,' First Girlfriend was saying. She stared intently at the undecipherable screen. Whatever she was doing down my gullet was more than uncomfortable. Jet lag, that's uncomfortable. This was different, an unnatural halfway house between pain and nausea.

I decided I was definitely in hell; that masturbation was a mortal sin after all. Who would've guessed? A hand pressed gently down on my shoulder but I couldn't see who it was, only the ominous shadow of its owner projected on the far wall. Then the camera settled in my stomach and once again my mind began to drift.

Martha and I went on holiday to the Amalfi coast. We sat at a bar with a glass of Prosecco, gazed over the blue sea far below as the sun set, and listened to an Italian crooner sing of love somewhere in the village. A breeze pushed cool, salty air around us, but there was no escape. From the outside we were just another couple, relaxing quietly on a Mediterranean terrace at the end of a day. Inside we wondered why Woe constantly sat next to us, sipping a Martini Rosso, humming along to something that sounded suspiciously like 'It's Now or Never'.

'What about a dog?' Martha brought up the pet thing again.

'No dogs.'

'A puffin? You still seem obsessed with them.'

'How do you know that?' I said.

'Internet history,' she replied. Was nothing sacred? Sadly, there were no puffin colonies on the Amalfi coast.

'We could,' Martha said later, as we walked home in the twilight, down the pebbled alleyway, past the lemon trees, 'try another woman's egg.'

'You can do that?' I asked, genuinely surprised. Martha nodded.

What kind of egg would we steal? I wondered. Blonde, Nordic, not too tall, intelligent but not quite as intelligent as Martha? Or maybe a brunette, or could you combine the two? Or Persian. Maybe we could have a half-Persian child. Imagine the bone structure on that...

'Or another man's sperm?'

I stopped. I saw some other guy's sperm getting it off with my wife's eggs. Some other dirty little latecomer inserted into the artificial penis, impregnating the woman I loved; the woman who I had wooed, wined and dined, and then proposed to.

'I wouldn't call it wooing,' Martha objected.

'I did woo you,' I replied, the other man's sperm now languishing in a pair of Speedos, enjoying the luxury of my wife's reproductive tracts.

'You gave me a Ferrero Rocher and felt me up in a park,' Martha sighed.

'That was wooing!'

Martha touched my cheek. Then, checking herself, she pulled it away.

'Roo,' she said. 'We might not be able to have a baby.'

Night fell. I tried to imagine a baby which was half Martha and half not me. I imagined our high-quality, illegal-sperm-based, six-foot-five Adonis of a son, walking off Centre Court at Wimbledon, on his way to finish a seminal paper on the cure for cancer.

'Dad,' he would say, placing his perfectly formed hand on my frail, elderly shoulder. 'There's something I've got to ask you.'

'Yes,' I would cry. 'It's true. You're not my son. We got you from a Jamaican physicist who won five gold medals in the Winter Olympics but had a gambling addiction...'

'What?'

'You know, the Winter Olympics? The ones that no one watches. There's the slalom...'

I stopped. I looked up at my slightly shocked not-quite-flesh-and-blood.

'Gee, Dad,' he said, 'I was just wondering what you wanted for your birthday.'

'Adoption?' Martha said.

The cicadas began to sing to each other. There it was. The final end point. A child completely unrelated to us, someone who was not ours at all. I went blank – could I love someone that wasn't my own flesh and blood? What if, by some chance, Martha got pregnant later on – could we love them both equally? Would it ever feel real? And if it did, what if they decided to reject you? I imagined my sixteen-year-old adopted Mongolian son looking down at me.

'Sorry, Dad, but it's something I've got to do.'

'Please don't. We can ferment milk here...'

'It's cow's milk, Dad, I need a yak's udder. I need to live in a yurt with my people...'

Tears in my eyes as I waved goodbye to my only child...

'Is there anything you are willing to do?' Martha finally gave up and went inside.

We discussed other things that might take the place of a child, hoping it would relieve some of the pressure, give us some other kind of home for our hopes, but the opposite happened: our desire for offspring grew more and more overbearing, with everything else pushed to the edges.

'What's happening to us?' Martha asked later that night as we lay in the dark, but the universe was silent. Then, the next morning, I started to bleed. A week later, back in London, I loosened my trousers in front of the doctor. His finger made a cursory inspection.

'You know,' he said, the finger going in a little deeper. 'You don't need to bring your wife every time you come to see me.'

'What is it?' I asked, ignoring him. I was keeping Martha close. He pulled out, snapped off the glove and started washing his hands.

'Not sure, but bleeding isn't good. How long has the weight loss been going on?'

I told him. The doctor rolled his eyes.

'You do realise this is why men die younger than women.'

I could die? As in dead? As in being dead? For the first time the possibility hit me. My life could just end. Bowel cancer. Run over by a bus. Attacked by a flightless bird.

'I could die,' I told Martha.

'I could remarry,' she nodded, 'Someone fertile.'

Stupid Martha. Here I was, a man with a malfunctioning digestive system, and she was treating the whole thing as a sideshow.

'It's probably just stress,' she said.

'Stress!' I shouted. 'Me?'

'All right, haemorrhoids then. Maybe you've got haemorrhoids and they're stressed.'

Martha did not have a sympathetic bedside manner. She regarded illness as a moral weakness. It was no use dying in front of Martha, your heart had to actually stop before she would go and get you soup.

I carefully checked the flat for Campbell's cream of chicken, just in case. I was now confronted with the fact that I might not have my own family because I might not live long enough. Then there would be no child, not a natural child, not an artificial, adopted, halfway, robot or any-other-way child.

There would be nothing.

'Mark?'

I gagged. It was First Girlfriend and I was back in the dark room. The walls were now spinning slightly, making me feel nauseous. Mr Pedantry appeared in front of me, tutting.

'Horry,' I said. 'Hi mean horsy-ated...'

Mr Pedantry disappeared and I gagged again, closed my eyes, and reopened them to find the face of First Girlfriend pressed up against mine.

'Hey,' she said, her lips half an inch away. 'Recognise this?'

I looked around; she was holding something but I found it impossible to focus. Eventually she moved her hand underneath the flickering light of the screen.

Plastic. It was the plastic. First Girlfriend was holding two used condoms in her hand.

'Why,' she whispered, 'are you still wearing them?'

Then I was in the hospital waiting to have my bowels examined for imminent death. There had been no seminar this time but my innards knew what was coming. They had just been cleared out by industrial-strength drain-o laxatives and were now preparing for some kind of rectal assault.

I tried to talk to Martha, but she was waiting for a call from work.

'They're going to stick something up me,' I said, glancing around the reception. A sign above the toilet door said 'Out of Order'.

'Welcome to the club,' Martha nodded, staring at her BlackBerry.

'That's different,' I whispered. 'Something often gets stuck up there. This is virgin territory.'

'Really?' Martha scrolled through her emails. 'No experiments at school?'

'No,' I frowned. 'I didn't go to public boarding school in south-east England.'

Martha's phone rang.

'It's work,' she said.

'Fine,' I snapped. Who cared about work? 'Just don't put me in one of your storylines.'

'We don't do proctology,' she replied, her tone suggesting she saw me in another part of the hospital entirely. 'It's not sexy.'

Martha left to talk to her producer. Then the nurse called me, and then it began. I soon saw what Martha meant about this particular corner of the medical world; it was not sexy. You couldn't see the doctors of *Holby* or *ER* arguing about whether the junior intern was ready to perform a full colonoscopy.

'Give me another metre of cable, stat!'

'Don't be a fool. His bowels can't take anymore…'

Normally, I like people who take an interest in their work, but not that day. To have the intricate details of your own lower digestive system explained whilst the camera was *in situ* was pushing things too far.

'You see here,' the proctologist pointed at the screen, pushing another inch up me. I tried to make sense of the shadowy indecipherable blackness on the screen.

'Yerrsss,' I said, in pain, in fear, air and water being pumped the wrong way up my digestive system. What was I seeing? Cancer? A wilting bowel? Was I pregnant? Was I now, by some curse, the first man ever to get pregnant?

'You're not pregnant,' he said shaking his head. 'It all looks normal. Now there's a tricky corner coming so you might feel a little discomfort.'

A tricky corner? I gave an unmanly whimper as the camera turned sharply. What kind of human being got into proctology?

'So what do you want to do, young lad?'

'Dunno, what about a loony doctor?'

'You mean psychiatry?'

'That's the one.'

'Full up.'

'Really? I want to mess with people's heads? What's the nearest thing?'

'Well, you could do worse than sticking things up someone's arse...'

Suddenly I was back in the room with the tube down my mouth and First Girlfriend in front of me. She looked frustrated, annoyed. The music had now changed to something by Whitney Houston.

'Take off the condoms,' she said.

'Ahm not arring any hondoms,' I replied.

She rolled her eyes. Had we not both done double English at school? Could I not see what she was getting at it? She wasn't literally telling me to remove prophylactics from my penis, was she?

'A hetafor?' I asked.

First Girlfriend nodded, her meaning finally comprehended by her drugged-up First Boyfriend. She kissed me on the cheek and then patted it.

'Goodbye,' she smiled. 'And good luck.'

Then something was leaving my stomach, moving up through my gullet, my throat, and out of my mouth. Suddenly I was free, free of the cable, free to cough, to swallow, to breathe. Lights went on. First Girlfriend dissolved, morphing into a consultant holding an endoscopy camera. Around her the white walls, the nurse, all came in to focus.

I wasn't dead. I wasn't in hell, or in the Matrix trying to negotiate with the One or the Architect or that random French character they introduced in the second film for no reason. I was in Procedure Room 6 at the Royal London near Whitechapel.

I sat up. The message of First Girlfriend was clear. I hadn't been taking it seriously, this thing called a family. I had been hedging my bets, covering myself against a future that wasn't perfect and fair and generous. Believing fate and nature and medicine owed me a baby. They owed me nothing. If I wanted a family I was going to have to earn it.

The condoms were off. I was going to get Martha a child, whatever it took. I sat up, felt dizzy.

'Where...' I started. The nurse pushed me back down on the trolley.

'We're taking you into recovery.'

'Where's my wife?' I said.

That night, possibly still a bit high, I promised Martha I would do whatever it took to get us a baby. Foreign eggs, sperm, mechanical wombs, whatever. If we needed to use donkey jizz, a barrel and Spanish grape-crushers to create our offspring then...

'Roo,' Martha said. 'I get it.'

Two weeks later, while eating breakfast, my results arrived in the post.

'Told you it was haemorrhoids,' smiled Martha, looking at the letter. I rubbed my chin, my stubble manly, my top button undone.

'Now,' she continued, 'we've got an appointment at the clinic next week. You ready?'

I cracked my knuckles. I picked up my cricket bat. I was ready. It was time to kick some undead fertility ass.

'You're not taking the bat.' Martha shook her head. 'Now eat your granola.'

I ate my granola.

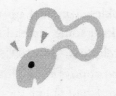

Chapter 17

One Last Stab at It

Come for lunch, Skelly x.

I read the text message, then put the phone back in my pocket. By my side was Martha; in front of me the undead Nurse Ratched. Silence surrounded us as we watched her bone-white fingers turn the pages of our notes, one by one.

'So,' she said, 'not pregnant then.'

'No,' we nodded.

'IVF was unsuccessful,' she continued. I didn't flinch. Let her state the obvious, let her try and wind me up; I had been to the underworld and survived. I was not taking any more nonsense from a zombie. At some stage I would still destroy her, all her kind, the clinic and possibly the free world, but first things first. I needed Nurse Ratched for the baby.

'No,' we agreed.

'I think,' her voice was soft, soothing, 'we should try embryo transfer.'

I smiled. Good old Nurse Ratched. Still predictable, still underestimating her opposition. This time, however, she was in for a surprise. I had spent the past weeks looking at options. I had read a book. Skimmed three pamphlets. From high-altitude sex to surrogate pregnancy, I was no longer the fledgling Luke Skywalker of the reproductive arts, but Lord Vader at the height of his powers, about to take charge of this fully functioning fertility Death Star.

'No,' I said.

Nurse Ratched looked up, surprised.

'Embryo transfer is the next step,' she said. 'We can't just rush into another cycle.'

My smile widened. Embryo transfer was not the next step. Embryo transfer was the next step for losers – it was just more IUI with embryos; and B grade embryos at that. I was no longer willing to just stroll along the yellow brick road of the St William's plan to not get us pregnant until we met the Wizard of Jizz...

And then Dorothy and The Scarecrow popped up, singing:

We're off to see the Jizzard,
The wonderful Jizzard of Oz.
We hear he is a whiz at jizz,
If ever some jizz there was...

'No,' I said.

Dorothy and The Scarecrow fell silent. Nurse Ratched pushed back with a volley of arguments. We had time to try a cycle of embryo transfer. The consultants would support her judgement, not ours, and she wasn't frightened of my assembled army of mixed-genre characters.

'Stop,' I raised my hand, sweeping away her protests. 'We only had two high-quality embryos and they didn't make it. The chances we'll get pregnant from the others can't be good. Anyway, they're frozen and we can still use them if the second try fails.'

I took a breath.

'We want IVF. We want to go again.'

The nurse stared at me, and then at Martha, as if somehow a staring competition with the wife would undermine us. I had no fear; Martha was a top-seeded starer and she wasn't going to blink. Not now. I waited for the inevitable.

'Very well,' Nurse Ratched tilted her head just a touch. 'We'll go for another round of IVF. We'll do the short protocol.'

'Short protocol?' I asked. 'There's a short protocol?'

'There is a protocol that's shorter,' she smiled, sensing a comeback.

Shorter?

'It takes less time,' Nurse Ratched continued as if explaining to a child. 'We do everything quicker.'

What was the point of the long protocol then? Why, when something could take less time, would you want it to take more? Why would they do that? The rage burned inside me and then...

... I stopped myself: it didn't matter, it was just the insane universe of reproductive medicine and soon it would all be destroyed. By the Death Star. By our baby.

Outside the clinic Martha pushed a prescription into my hand.

'Can you pick it up for me?' she asked.

I grabbed it, ready to do battle with The Troglodyte, but Martha shook her head.

'A normal chemist will have this.'

I gave the prescription to our pharmacist. He regarded it with confusion for a moment and then nodded.

'You'll need to pay for this,' he said.

'Don't I always?' I asked. I was already one of the three or four remaining people in the UK who had to pay for drugs.

'Not for the pill.' He shook his head. 'You only pay for the pill if you're trying to have a baby.'

I tapped a finger on the counter three times.

'The pill?' I asked.

'Yes, this is a prescription for the pill.'

'The contraceptive pill?'

'The contraceptive pill.'

I came home and threw the packet of Marvelon onto Martha's lap.

'The pill?' I asked.

She nodded.

'The pill helps you get pregnant?'

'Of course not,' Martha said. 'It stops me getting pregnant. They're using the pill to regulate my cycle.'

'Your cycles are regular! If they set up Ofcycle to regulate cycles, you'd be its Chief Executive...'

'It's not funny the eighteenth time,' Martha raised her voice.

What was this, a Grisham novel? All these perverse protocols? Was Jack Nicholson staring down at Tom Cruise, shouting: 'You want the pill? You can't handle the pill...'

The Death Star now appeared to be under attack from rebel forces. Again, I had underestimated the insane causal structure in the outer dimensions of reproductive medicine. Martha started to open the packet. What next? I wondered. A hysterectomy?

We went to Single Mike's for dinner. He greeted us at the door.

'You poor, poor creatures...'

'Michael,' I said.

'Mark,' he sniffed, slightly annoyed at his continuous eulogy being interrupted.

'Shut up.'

Single Mike sat me next to a particularly vitriolic woman.

'What about the children that die of cancer?'

I didn't care. About the woman, that is. I hoped one day to have a vested interest in children not dying of cancer or preferably just not getting cancer at all. Her statement didn't surprise me, though I did wonder how Mike managed to get so much information to his dinner guests about our problems. Did he have a blog?

'What *about* the children,' I repeated slowly, 'who die of cancer?'

'If we didn't have to pay for IVF they could get them the drugs, couldn't they?'

'Do you...' I slammed the table. All conversation stopped. '... have a child who's dying of cancer and being denied treatment? Because, if you do, I will give you the money. I will write a cheque now. I will go down to the hospital and steal the drugs.'

She stared at me, venom dripping from her home-made Vietnamese spring roll.

'Don't be facetious,' she said.

Facetious. Never use the word. Never think it will make you look eloquent or socially superior. It's been on *Coronation Street*. It's like shouting 'carpe diem' at an interview for the chair of Latin at Christchurch. It's embarrassing.

'Thank you,' I said to the woman, as if she'd offered me a compliment, and then we left Single Mike's for the last time.

The next day I went to a department store and brought several pairs of David Beckham-sponsored underwear a size too small. When Martha arrived home she found me in a pair, nursing a beer on my tummy, watching *The Genesis of the Daleks* on VHS.

'Attractive,' she said.

My newfound insights had led to further truths. Until this point I had made a begrudging attempt to follow the advice of fertility books, but I now realised they all had something in common: if you took their advice, you would die. They were just giant lists, hundreds of pages long, of things you can't do, all written by a puritan from the first American colonies who'd time-travelled into the twenty-first century and needed a book deal.

'So what are your areas of expertise?'

'Starvation, chastity and the vengeance of the Lord.'

'Mmm. Have you thought about writing about reproduction?'

We already knew that alcohol and cigarettes and caffeine were foetal Armageddon, but that wasn't enough for a book. That was a pamphlet. You can't sell a pamphlet. So the list went on:

peanuts were deadly, which makes you wonder about monkeys and Thailand. Mobile phones were equally fatal to womb-based existence, especially when one was placed on or near your genitals. Who would do that?

'Darling, what are you doing? Is that my iPhone?'
  'It's got a special app!'

Food is bad. All food. Don't go near electricity pylons, live in a city, town, or any other place inhabited by humans. Don't drive a car, become emotionally imbalanced, or have gas. If you feel unwell or flatulent whilst trapped in your unheated, isolated Scandinavian hut eating turnips, don't think about getting medical assistance. Here are the drugs one book suggested avoiding while trying to conceive:

  Antibiotics
  Antidepressants
  Antihistamines
  Antihypertensives
  Antimalarial pills
  Antiviral drugs
  Decongestants
  Inhalers
  NSAID painkillers
  Sleeping pills
  Steroids

Ironically, the pill didn't make it onto the list, but I guess that would be academic as you suffocated from an asthma attack after attempting a round of scheduled sex.

And yet ketamine addicts have babies. Rod Stewart has babies. Resistance fighters in occupied France, Egyptian slaves dragging stone blocks across the desert, starving medieval peasants during the Black Death – they all somehow still managed to reproduce. Health and well-being don't seem to have much to do with it.

So the books went in the bin. Not the recycling bin, but the proper one. I wasn't taking any chances. Relaxed, I sipped my beer and Martha curled in next to me and we bathed in the child-killing rays of the TV together.

With the Death Star now hovering above the planet Hubris, we went around to Ms Skeletor's for lunch. Her home, a small two-bedroom garden flat, was nicely done in the mid-century style and, glass of wine in hand, she gave us the brief tour; the living room, the little kitchen with a tiny walled garden, the bathroom, the main bedroom, the second bedroom...

the child's bed. Martha and I took a sudden intake of breath. It was so neatly made up, the sheets so clean and fresh, the little shelf on the opposite wall full of unread children's books. A toy box.

It was our second bedroom. If we'd conceived all those years ago, in the honeymoon suite of that hotel with the fish, this was how it would look. It was our life if things had turned out as planned.

We turned to Ms Skeletor. Was she insane? Was the room a shrine to a child never conceived? Were we now in the hands of a broken woman who would soon try to convince us that little non-existent Bobby or Oliver or Sarah was just staying at a friend's and due home any day soon?

'I'm not mad,' Ms Skeletor laughed, seeing our faces. 'I'm adopting.'

The glass in her hand shook ever so slightly, but her eyes sparkled in the dim light of the basement flat. Soon, they said, soon their gaze would fall upon a child of her own. All that trapped love, desperate to be released, sensing freedom was near.

'Congratulations,' said Martha, looking at Ms Skeletor intensely, curious. Then we went out into the light of the kitchen and talked media and drank a wine spritzer and ate something by Jamie Oliver.

And then, later, as night fell, Martha and I finally arrived at the worst fight in the world, triggered by those simple words accompanied by tears. The worst words in the world.

'I just,' Martha said, crying, 'want a baby.'

Marriage. It's not simple. One minute you're in it together; destroying undead nurses and struggling with condoms and going through the menopause. The next you're heading towards divorce. I often threaten to end our marriage when Martha is being unreasonable, but that night, five minutes post the worst words in the universe, I truly wanted everything to end.

'You want a divorce?' Martha shouted.

'Damn right. I'm ringing my lawyer tomorrow.'

'You don't have a lawyer.'

I considered this. There was that woman who did our flat.

'She was a conveyancing solicitor.'

Couldn't she multitask?

'And what would you do after the divorce?' Martha was suddenly all pretend-calm.

The annoying thing about Martha is, in a fight, she tries to make you think about things. Tries to appear logical. Says the word 'narrative' a lot. I didn't want to think about things or be logical, and the narrative was that I was a saint and my wife was the most frustrating woman on the planet.

'Well?'

I thought about it. I thought I would probably miss Martha very much. I thought I wouldn't be very happy and who would commentate over the News so I couldn't actually hear what was going on in the world? Who would cook hamburgers?

'Maybe you're right,' she continued, now horrifyingly calm. 'Maybe we should end this. An amicable divorce.'

She held out a trembling hand to shake on the matter. Then came the pesto pasta, the bath and the tears and that's what you get when you don't start a fight on a Saturday morning in an orderly fashion.

Then I was back in St William's, argument over, my penis pointing optimistically towards the ceiling. Then I was shuffling out of the anti-wank chair, handing in my specimen, and sitting down next to Martha amongst the infertile throng.

'Martha Cossey,' a nurse called out. Martha gripped my hand and led me into the ward. At that moment both of us felt that neither God nor man could give us a baby.

They came for Martha. After she was pushed away, I walked out of the clinic. One more thing needed to be done. I went down to the ground floor, out of the building and onto the busy street. I found a corner to stand on and took a small rectangular box out of my pocket. I opened the flap.

I took out a single cigarette, tar content 1.6 mg, and waved it at the heavens. It was my offering, my one finger up to all the mediation-loving, peanut-fearing, IUI-worshiping fools. I took out a match, lit it, and drew deeply. A light dizziness hit me and I prayed silently, prayed to whoever would listen:

This time, just this time, I prayed. The Death Star aimed its weapon at the planet Hubris.

'Sorry, mate,' a voice said, 'can I ponce a fag?'

To my right was a small man. He was carrying several copies of *The Big Issue* and his bloodshot eyes looked up at me like a lost dog.

I considered his unwashed hair, his stubble, the new trainers with the laces missing. He was someone's son. He had once been conceived, born, the cord cut, a mother's arm picking him up and embracing him. Then what? Where had it gone wrong? Had he been abandoned, orphaned, abused? Or did things just sometimes not work out?

I handed him the packet. He began to extract a single cigarette.

'Take them,' I said.

'Really?' he smiled.

'Go on.'

'Thanks, mate,' he said. 'Thanks a lot.'

He walked away. I took a final drag, threw the cigarette in the gutter and stood for a moment, swaying slightly from the nicotine rush. Then I went back to the clinic.

In recovery Martha was sleeping. Eight eggs had been collected in the harvest. There was nothing to do but go home and wait for the call telling us how many embryos were produced and what quality they were.

We sat down for dinner. I looked across at Martha, expecting her to be engrossed in her food. Instead I found her staring back at me, a small tear trying to escape from the corner of her eye. She stretched out her hand and placed it, palm down on the table.

'Will we be OK?' she asked.

I understood. Were we going to be OK without kids for the rest of our lives? Something so fundamental had broken many couples, undermined many a marriage; would it do the same to us? For a moment there was a vacuum. A nothingness. Then, underneath all the noise of a relationship, all the commitments and shared memories and friends and things, the nub of it came to me.

I realised I loved my wife.

It should have been the most obvious thing in the world; a husband loving his wife. Perhaps it had been so clear that I had never questioned it, looked it in the face to check it was still there. Either that or there's the remotest possibility that I may, in some things, emotional things, be just the slightest bit slow.

I put my hand on Martha's. If it ended up just the two of us, watching *University Challenge* with a stuffed puffin on the sideboard, then so be it. That was more than enough. There was only one answer to her question:

'Boo,' I said.

'Yes?'

'It'll be fine.'

Martha gave me the smallest of smiles. Her hand turned over and our fingers intertwined. For once, her husband knew what he was talking about. Then we ate our dinner.

The next day we discovered, for the second time, that our embryos were excellent, which proved that, if we did ever have a baby, it would clearly be winning awards in the field of excellence. Martha, susceptible as ever to the power of a compliment, beamed sheepishly when she told me:

'He said that one of the embryos was an A star.'

I raised an eyebrow.

'There's an A star?'

'Yep – it's even better than an A.'

Better than an A. I tried to be positive, but it really doesn't matter how excellent your embryos are, or how ugly other people's babies are. They still have their ugly babies and you're still stuck with your excellent embryos.

We went back to the clinic on Wednesday and someone must have died, or finally gone insane, because, instead of whale music or the pan pipes, we had hits from the Baroque. To the tune of 'Zadok the Priest', which would certainly give our unborn child an overstated sense of their own importance, Geoffrey placed two of our most excellent embryos back in to Martha's most excellent uterus.

'Now, I don't need to tell you,' said the nurse handing us a pregnancy test, 'you must wait the full two weeks. Two weeks.'

We nodded. We swung out of the clinic and headed back to work. I didn't allow myself to feel anything. I dared not. I promised myself that I was not even going to consider the possibility of a pregnancy. I had buried hope in the deepest hole I could find and poured concrete on it.

Ten days in, we got up as normal. Martha paced in front of the toilet door as I got ready for work.

'Just do the test when you're ready,' I said.

'No, no, I'll wait the full two weeks.'

'Only if you want to.'

'I'll wait.'

I got as far as the tube station when the phone rang. It was Martha.

'I couldn't wait,' her voice trembled down the line. I took a breath, closed my eyes, ready to hear that most familiar word. The word which had been repeated exactly forty-five times in our search for a baby.

'It's...' *Negative*, I thought. '... positive.'

'What?'

'It's positive. I think I'm pregnant.'

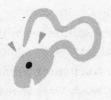

Chapter 18

The Grain of Rice

This is how I pictured it. Some slow-motion camera work, a montage of me in various heroic situations: slaying a dragon, downing a Messerschmitt, knocking out middle stump. The winning ace for game, set and match, the defused bomb, the blue lightsaber still over the black robes. Martha appears. We slap high fives and dance around the flat to the tune of 'Xanadu'. The ELO version, not the Olivia Newton-John one. Friends and family join us in a giant bear hug as magnums, nay jeroboams and nebuchadnezzars, of champagne are sprayed over us, everyone crying with joy and relief as we all dance down our suddenly pedestrianised street towards Wembley stadium or the O2 arena, gradually joined by Marv, the German Cockney doctor, the Italian consultant, Geoffrey the embryologist, the undead Nurse Ratched, Nurse Mime, The Wicked Witch, Dorothy, The Scarecrow, the Morgans, Single Mike, Darwin, Paxman, The Gremlin, The Troglodyte, a flock of puffins, some antibodies, the pigeons and millions of pink sperm; confetti being thrown out the windows of London by millions of well-wishers...

That's how I imagined it. Instead:

'Fuck,' I said.

I started to run. Unaccustomed as I am to running, I fell over almost immediately, scraping my arm against the pavement. It began to bleed. Someone tried to help me up but I pushed them away and charged off again, men and women of the city parting in front of me, creating a human pathway to my home. Then I was bounding up the stairs and finally pushing the key into the lock and swinging the door open. Then I stood there, bloody and breathless, in front of Martha, the woman whom I, along with several others who had dedicated their life to reproductive medicine, had finally gotten pregnant.

I stared at her.

'Fuck,' I said.

Martha presented me with the testing stick. I studied it. I realised I had never really looked at a test before and had no idea which part of it showed proof of the pregnancy.

'The double blue line.' Martha pointed at two thin strips.

There it was: two faint, blue lines, proof of the beginnings of life. They looked so fragile, those strips of blue; so likely to be wrong, so unconvincing, this first indicator that Martha was now with child.

'Fuck,' I said.

'I've done three already,' Martha bit her nails.

What was there to say? How did she retain that amount of urine?

I sat down. We couldn't get too excited; these tests were only ninety-eight billion per cent accurate.

'We can't get too excited,' I said.

'No,' Martha agreed.

'It could be a false positive,' I said.

'Do you know what that means?' Martha asked. I did not.

'Or a phantom pregnancy?' I continued to explore the options. Could it be a phantom pregnancy? I imagined a ghostly presence in Martha's womb.

'Shut up now,' Martha took the test back off me, but I needed to say something. Some kind of powerful emotion was welling up inside me.

'We need to keep calm.' I stood up and paced around our living room, but the feeling continued its ascent. I expected it to burst into relief, happiness, the purity of a test century, the divine contentment of Constantine the Great when the true God was revealed to him.

But it was nothing like that. This was something else, something new.

What?

'Fear,' Martha answered.

Spot on as always. It was fear. A new kind of fear. Suddenly we were terrified, not for ourselves or for each other, but for that tiniest sliver of existence that was taking its first tentative steps towards life inside Martha's tummy.

Would it survive? Could it?

Over the next four days Martha used up our cold-war-sized stockpile of test kits, continuing to reassure ourselves that she was still pregnant. We fretted: we removed all alcohol, hot water, unpasteurised cheese, peanuts and other menaces from the house. We charcoaled our meat with a blowtorch. I spent my time phoning Martha, making sure she was relaxed, calm. Eventually she stopped picking up, which was stressful.

'At least we can keep it to ourselves,' I said, listening to Martha's liver for signs of the baby.

'How so?' she replied, putting down the Christmas edition of *Kitchen and Bathroom*.

'Everyone keeps it a secret for the first three months,' I said. It was the rule: you don't announce until after the twelve-week scan.

Martha sighed, lifted my head off her internal organs, and got up. She brought over the laptop and opened Facebook.

'See that.' She pointed to the number of friends we had in common. It was eighty-seven.

'My God,' I said.

'Exactly...' Martha began.

'Cricket's devil number. We have the unluckiest number of mutual friends possible.'

'... not what I meant at all,' she finished. 'Right now eighty-seven people, plus anyone who's been to Single Mike's for dinner over the past eighteen months, are going to want to know whether we're up the duff in about...'

Martha paused to look at my watch.

'... seven days ago.'

I looked at Martha's Facebook page. Was this so bad? She was, after all, pregnant now. She'd been pregnant for almost three weeks, surely it was time to break out the champagne, do a little dance, make a little social love. Burn some things.

'Roo,' Martha looked at me. 'You do know why people wait twelve weeks to announce it, don't you?'

I stared at her, unsure. Tradition?

'Miscarriage,' Nurse Ratched said a day later.

Minutes before I had been a happy father-to-be. We had sat down with the Ratched. She made Martha do another test, and then, examining the stick, looked at us and nodded.

'Positive,' she said.

'But not false positive?' I asked, anxiously.

'Shut up,' she replied, sensing that she might finally be rid of my presence. Suddenly, in a moment of clarity I wondered whether to Nurse Ratched we were the undead. The souls in need of salvation. She leaned towards Martha and gave her two embarrassed, tentative pats on the knee.

'You're pregnant.'

Yee-ha! I forgot about undead relativism as applied to Ratched. The only way was up and you couldn't stop us now. We were going to have a baby! We were going to be a family; I was going to be a paterfamilias at last. Mentally, I started doing the samba. Suddenly I was strutting my Latin moves across the dance stage of Belgium's biggest Latin dance festival. I don't know why I was doing that. If ever there were two cultures that didn't mix they were a bunch of geeky Flemish youths trying to groin-thrust each other Latin-style in a pile of mud somewhere in Flanders...

'Now, about the chances of a miscarriage,' Nurse Ratched continued.

The muddy, beer-strewn festival floor was whipped from under me. Miscarriage? Why was anyone talking about miscarriage? My experiences with *EastEnders* had taught me all I thought I'd ever need to know about miscarriage: it was always brought on by being kicked in the stomach, falling down stairs or drinking vodka. As we lived in a single-storey flat, preferred gin, and I wasn't flexible enough to land a foot on Martha's midriff, I assumed we were OK.

'The chances are somewhere between ten and twenty per cent for any pregnancy.' Nurse Ratched's voice was all sweetness and light.

I slumped into my chair. The undead. There was always a twist in the tale whenever you dealt with the undead.

'You shouldn't worry.' She smiled.

Worry? Ten to twenty per cent and we're not to worry? We'd come all this way and now there was a one-in-five chance of it not happening? I'd brought the holy water and the garlic and now we might have a miscarriage?

We walked out of St William's. It would be another three weeks before a scan would show anything, twenty-one days before we'd know what was happening inside Martha's womb.

God, I pleaded, *please don't let Martha miscarry*. Think of the puffins.

The weeks passed in a sort of emotional wasteland. We tried hard not to engage with the little person growing away. Martha tried not to order a buggy, a cot, the nappies. I tried not to rehearse my brilliant dad jokes.

'I'm off now,' I'd say, in some imagined future, to my fine offspring, all lined up by the front door to bid their father goodbye. 'Some say I've been off for years.'

Much hearty laughter from my brood of healthy youngsters. Then later, playing canasta after supper, I might slam my cards on the table.

'This hand's so bad it's a foot!'

Peals of joy from my progeny, the mirth never stopping in the Cossey household. From the classic 'let's make like a guillotine and head off' to the subtle 'you're not quite a wit, but you're halfway there', I dreamt of an audience, too young to take out a restraining order, related by blood, enraptured by my punning time and time again.

Finally it came. The day of the scan, the day that would give us ultimate proof that what was inside Martha was a growing, potential baby. Christmas was everywhere now, the weather cold, the decorations up in every shop and office, the restaurants full, their festive menus on a board outside. We walked past the ancient church of St Anne.

I felt sick. A stone sat in my stomach.

We found ourselves in a new room, more spacious, with enough space even for all of us to sit comfortably. We had been upgraded to the upper-class lounge of the clinic.

The doctor began to chat. I love the chat. Who wouldn't want to make some small talk, to fiddle around with a bit of bureaucracy? We'd waited four years to get this first view of our baby, we didn't know if it was alive or dead, but what the hell – let's have a chat. We'll have a look later. After all, she'd already seen a dozen foetuses that morning so what's the rush?

'Is this your name?' she asked Martha, pointing at Martha's name on a form. No, of course it wasn't. We'd kidnapped the real Martha to steal her ultrasound slot. We were actually Sri Lankan health tourists with surprisingly fair skin and excellent London accents.

'And how are you feeling?' the consultant continued her inquiries, running a finger along lines in the notes.

Impatient to see our baby!

Finally, the chat ended. Martha got onto a trolley. I had been to an ultrasound before so I wasn't surprised when the doctor pulled out a device that looked like a giant dildo. The shock came when it turned out to actually be a giant dildo.

'Now,' the doctor said, slapping on some latex gloves and covering the dildo in goo. 'I'm going to put this inside you and we are going to have a look.' With dildo-cam inserted into Martha and her hand grasping mine in fear and discomfort, the three of us went off in search of our baby. This was it: the scan would tell us if there really, truly was something growing inside. Weird images started to appear on the TV screen attached to the camera, and the doctor studied them intently.

And silently.

Ultrasounds are to medicine what James Joyce novels are to literature. It's not clear what's going on but everyone tries to tell you how important it is. My eyes strained to see something in the mass of static that morphed this way and that, but I could make out nothing. Panic reeled through me: maybe there was nothing, nothing at all. And to think everyone laughed at my phantom pregnancy diagnosis! Well, no one's laughing now, are they? No one's laughing now.

Then the doctor stopped, holding the camera in a specific position for what seemed like an eon. I can't avoid stating the obvious: it was a pregnant pause. It literally was a pause while we waited to find out whether we were truly pregnant or not. The doctor tilted her head, we tilted ours. The doctor peered closer into the monitor. We peered with her. She went 'Mmmm'.

'Excuse me,' I finally said.

'Mmm?' The doctor's eyes remained fixed on the screen as her right hand started to once again move the camera around Martha's innards. What could we possibly want to know?

'The baby?'

The doctor kept moving, as if unsure which baby we were talking about.

'You want to know about your baby?' she asked.

What other knowledge could we possibly want? Who really constructed the pyramids? Is murder ever justified? Martha was on the edge of tears. It was beyond reason that we should wait any longer. I stared at the doctor and then at the screen but neither was giving anything away. Was I going to scream?

'Yes,' I pleaded. 'We just want to know about our baby.'

The doctor stopped again, allowing the image to settle on some unknown region of Martha's reproductive system. The senseless ultrasound static continued to reveal nothing.

Then she turned to us.

'Look.'

She pressed a button, and there, in the sea of grey, a tiny pulse of red appeared. Then it pulsed again. And again and again. A little red beacon signalling to us from Martha's womb.

'That,' the doctor said, 'is your baby's heartbeat.'

I'm not a spiritual man, but at that moment I died and went to heaven. Oblivion threw its soft blanket around me and I fell into its embrace, my existence complete, the job of life finally done, the universe shrunk down to that one little red pulse, beating in the static.

'Mark,' a voice called. The universe returned.

'Mark,' Martha called again, her eyes fixed on the red pulse. 'We're having a baby.'

Tears swelled in my eyes. Martha's hand tightened around mine. For the first time it hit me. Yes, there was still fear, fear for that little heartbeat, fear for the mother that would have to carry it, fear for myself, but suddenly mixed in was a joy, the single greatest joy ever known to humanity.

The joy of our own little heartbeat.

'It's about the size of a grain of rice,' the doctor shrugged, not helping the moment. We didn't care. It was our grain of rice and it had a beat. Wiping tears from my eyes, I found Martha a tissue, helped her off the trolley, and we sat down next to one another for one last chat with the doctor.

'What now?' Martha asked.

'Book yourself in to see your GP. They'll talk you through it.'

'We don't need to come back?'

'Not for this baby – you're normal now.'

Normal. We were normal. The greatest sentence ever invented. After four long, hard years we were normal. A tinge of guilt hit me as we walked out through the waiting room, all puffy-eyed and normal; I could see everyone feel sorry for us and all we could do was silently wish them all a heartbeat, a heartbeat that was worth a lifetime's wait.

Outside the sun had arrived, London was busy being London. We took a moment and let the world move around us.

'How do you feel?' I asked.

Martha considered the question. How did she feel? Scared? Happy? Relieved?

'Pregnant,' she said. 'I feel pregnant.'

We embraced. Standing between the hospital, the church and the pub we kissed. We had done it. Without doubt that little heartbeat was going to scare us; what was growing inside Martha was a future child that would laugh, play, get angry, eat peanuts in Thailand, do however many thousands of terrifying and beautiful things.

We weren't at the end at all. We were just slightly late for the beginning.

Martha patted her stomach and then looked at my watch.

'We'd better get on,' she said, preparing new lists in her head. There was so much to be done!

But we paused a moment longer, side by side. Then, the winter sun low in the sky and the world anew, the three of us walked off into the city. A family.

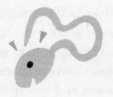

Epilogue

You Never Really Make It

Thirty-six weeks later, on Jimmy's due date, Martha and I were in an ambulance, getting lost.

'You're going the wrong way,' she screamed, as another set of contractions began. I knew I was supposed to be timing something but exactly what escaped me.

The driver shot me a smile.

'If I had a fiver for every time a woman told me that,' he winked. I shook my head in pity; the poor man was dead.

We stopped at a red light on the Mile End Road. I stood aside; allowing my wife to turn, get the driver in her sights and talk him through the best route through London's notoriously complicated road system.

'Turn around,' she said, butterflies and faeries carrying her gentle words to the driver.

'It's a one-way system, love, we...'

Martha looked confused. Were we not in an emergency vehicle? Did we not have power over all roads?

'Turn,' she screamed. 'The fuck. Around. *Now*.'

The driver turned. Then the contractions really kicked in and the satnav began to work and the ambulance's siren started to wail. Ten minutes later we passed our flat, again, Martha belting out directions.

'Not Aldersgate,' she bellowed. 'What use is Aldersgate? Where do you think we're having this baby? Scotland?'

It was 3.30 in the afternoon and things were moving at a speed no one had expected.

Our own preparation for the birth had been patchy. We had, for example, not finished our birthing plan. Birthing plans are a way of allowing every mother-to-be to let the hospital staff know how they would like to be treated, and what little things would help make the birth special for them. This allows the hospital to add disappointment to a list of emotions the mother would feel on the day.

'Ah, Mrs Sucker, your plan says you want to give birth in a pool of yak's milk with Wagner's 'Ride of the Valkyries' performed on a ukulele and four sticks of triple-amber incense lit the moment the baby comes out?'

'Yep.'

'Brilliant. Nurse, dope her up and prep the theatre.'

We were further unprepared by the antenatal course we did before the birth. It was terrible. It was like the Pope giving you advice about the wedding night. The woman running it had a way about her, a descriptive turn of phrase that convinced me birth was like the film *Saw*, except it was actually going to happen. To Martha.

'We're going to do drugs,' I said. 'Lots of drugs.'

The woman tutted. She explained how all drugs given in a hospital maternity wing were basically forms of legalised child abuse and any woman who went for something stronger than paracetamol was not fit to be a mother.

If men gave birth, it would go like this:

'Giving birth?'

'Yep.'

'Right. Nurse, some whisky, heroin, then a general anaesthetic and an epidural. That OK for you?'

'Dunno. I do really feel pain…'

The antenatal woman sensed my uncertainty about a drug-free birth.

'You know what the greatest drug in the world is?' she asked.

Nicotine? Methadone? It depended on your criteria of 'great'.

'Two words,' she said. 'Two words are all you need to remember.'

Everyone waited to hear this inspirational couplet, this incantation that would guide our partners painlessly through childbirth.

'Calm down,' she said, her hands pushing gently down on imaginary shoulders. '"Calm down" is what you tell her.'

The men of the class collectively raised their eyebrows. Calm down? I still had scars from the last time I told Martha to calm down, and that was because her hair had been dyed the wrong colour. You're better off admitting a long-standing affair with your wife's sister than telling her to calm down during labour.

'We'll stick with drugs,' I replied, calming down.

Then, on the twenty-fourth of July, it happened. Martha was on the phone, trying to convince me to do some nesting. She wanted, of all things, a clock from Dwell.

'Dwell?' What was this new place for a domestic dispute?

'Yes, Dwell,' Martha replied. 'You've vetoed IKEA and Habitat. Our choices are limited.'

I was suspicious of Dwell. For starters, humans don't dwell. They live, they doss down, they reside, but they don't dwell. Goblins dwell. Maybe the store was run by a horde of goblins.

'It's not run by goblins,' Martha sighed. I began to think of the goblins.

'Right,' said the goblin CEO of Dwell, 'we've got to offload all this imitation mid-century furniture we stole during our conquests of Scandinavia in the 1960s.'

'We could set up a chain selling it to the humans for their dwellings.'

'Good thought, Spinnbarkeit, but what would we call it?'

Dwell is a negative word. People only dwell on bad things that happened in the past. No one dwells optimistically. You're never going to hear the phrase: '"One day I'll have my own dwelling to dwell in," he dwelled hopefully.'

'The clock, Boo,' Martha cut in. I agreed to get the clock and hung up. Then my phone rang again.

'I'm getting it,' I said.

'Will you come home?' Martha's voice sounded less clock-obsessed now.

'Are you OK?'

'Fine. I just feel, well, odd.'

'Contractions?'

'Maybe, I don't know…'

My wife is many things, but stoic in the face of pain isn't one of them. We had confirmed that whatever happened, from the moment we walked into the hospital, we wanted at least an epidural, ideally a caesarean, or better still a surrogate to actually have the baby. We certainly weren't going to muck about with some hippy nonsense like a birthing pool and more whale music.

So if Martha was only feeling 'odd', I was sure things were fine. Even her waters were intact. Still, it couldn't hurt if I came home and relieved her mum for a bit.

I got to the flat. Martha wanted some chocolate so I went back out to the store and brought her a Flake. When I got back she was in the loo. I waited a minute, but she didn't come out. Hairs pricked up on the back of my neck.

'Are you OK?' I called out.

There was no answer, but the door opened, and I heard Martha go back into our bed. I followed her – she was looking more worried now.

'Can you have a look in the toilet?' she said, waving me away.

There was blood in the bowl. Not masses, but not spotting either. I knew blood could be either normal or not, so what was I looking for? How much blood was bad? Why doesn't the NCT teach you anything useful? As it dispersed in with the water I realised I had no idea what it signified. Then Martha cried out.

'Roo,' she cried. 'Roo.'

I raced into the bedroom. Martha was now breathing heavily and lying in a substantial pool of blood. This, I knew, was not normal at all. No waters broken, no obvious contractions how could she be bleeding like this? Her eyes, wide open, pleaded with me to tell her that it was OK. I took a deep breath. *Keep calm*, I told myself.

'I'll call an ambulance,' I said, rushing into the hall. I picked up the phone – it was time to man up, I told myself, trembling as I punched the three numbers into the phone. Time to stay in control, to get help to my wife as quickly as possible.

Then a voice started talking in my ear:

'The number you have dialled has not been recognised...'

I realised the voice was coming from the phone.

I dialled the emergency services again. Again the same message. What had happened? How could the emergency services be down? Had there been a terrorist attack? Had civilisation collapsed? The key thing was not to panic.

'It's down!!' I shouted. 'I can't get through!'

'What number did you call?' Martha cried from the bedroom. She was now in a lot of pain.

I stopped and thought for a minute.

'Nine,' I said.

'And?'

I felt slightly foolish.

'And?'

'One,' I mumbled.

'And.'

'One,' I said, but only to myself.

Stupid Hollywood.

I punched 9 9 9. Within seconds I was through to the ambulance service, and with encouragement from Martha screaming in the background, help arrived in the form of a nice paramedic on a bicycle.

'How is she?' asked the lycra-clad medic.

'Probably not well enough to travel by bike,' I replied.

Then Martha's mother turned up and the next thing I knew, we were going the wrong way up the Mile End Road towards proctology.

Thirty minutes later, we finally arrived at the correct hospital. All attempts to measure Martha's contractions had been in vain – they seemed way too close together for someone who had started labour less than an hour before. The crew got her out of the ambulance and in a second we had stormed our way up to the third floor of the maternity wing.

This was unfortunate as it was the wrong floor. The third floor was prenatal and for several minutes a lot of expectant mothers, waiting for their twelve-week scan, got a first-hand look at exactly what was going to happen to them.

'The second floor!' Martha cried. The ambulancemen looked at me a little sheepishly.

'We're from Bromley,' they said, frantically pressing the down button.

We arrived in the birthing unit. There was no time for pools or your favourite CD or a birth plan. The midwife took one look at Martha and the next thing we knew we were in a room, Martha kneeling on the bed, screaming her heart out.

I held her arms. Having vaguely listened to the NCT classes on childbirth, I knew what lay ahead. Hours, days perhaps, of labour, swearing, tears, insults – and that would just be me confronting the medical staff to get my wife an aspirin. Clutching her hand tightly, I steadied my legs; this was it, I thought, this was when the man walks out to the wicket, checks his guard and makes sure his family gets every, little, thing that it needs. Makes sure that…

'That's its head!' cried the midwife.

What? Whose head? Where were the hours of painful contractions?

'One more push,' cried the nurse. What about the gas, the pethidine, the needle in the spine? What about the traditional British emergency caesarean which no one saw coming?

'Hang on,' the midwife looked momentarily confused, then she smiled. 'Ah, he's still in his amniotic sac.'

'What?'

'He's still in his caul – look.'

The little fellow had come out in a bubble. That's why Martha's waters hadn't broken; our first child had been born inside them.

'Is that bad?' I asked, fretful. 'Will he drown?'

'It's good luck,' laughed the midwife, 'it's a one-in-a-thousand thing. I've only seen it a few times.'

Then she added:

'Except in Bulgaria, where it means he's a vampire.'

On that note she burst the caul, and seconds later we heard a sound that we were going to have to get used to. For the first time our baby began to cry.

'Do you want to hold him?' the nurse asked Martha.

Later that night, we were all on the ward. For some reason we had been given our own room, perhaps as a reward for having the fastest labour ever. Martha was eating a samosa, I was sitting in an easy chair, holding our four-hour-old boy close. Outside, other babies were crying. Lots of babies.

'Roo,' Martha smiled at me.

'Boo,' I said, smiling back.

'Jimmy,' she said. 'What about "Jimmy"?'

I looked down at my boy, his eyes shut, his lips puckering, his whole body unsure of itself.

'Jimmy,' I nodded. Now he had a name and now we were what we'd always wanted to be. A family. We had everything in the world in that little room. We were complete. I began to drift off.

'You know what?' Martha said, her eyes closing.

'What?'

'We need another baby.' Then she dozed off.

My eyes popped open. Another? I sat in the chair with Jimmy. Since we'd first turned the lights off all those years ago, I had never, even for an instant, counted past one.

I looked down at Jimmy. I realised, in the cool hospital air, with my wife and son asleep, that things weren't over at all. That what we'd been through was nothing compared to what was to come. Martha was right; the little baby I was holding would need a partner in crime, a companion on life's journey, and his parents would do anything to make that happen. Soon, we were going to have to go through it all again.

And so we did.

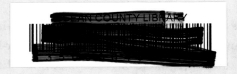

Have you enjoyed this book?
If so, why not write a review on your favourite website?

If you're interested in finding out more about our books,
find us on Facebook at **Summersdale Publishers** and follow
us on Twitter at **@Summersdale**.

Thanks very much for buying this Summersdale book.

www.summersdale.com